Lipids:
A Clinicians' Guide

Lipids:
A Clinicians' Guide

Leon A. Simons* and Joyce Corey Gibson†

* Senior Lecturer in Medicine, University of New South Wales; Physician-in-charge Lipid Clinic, St. Vincent's Hospital Sydney, and Director Sydney Coronary Heart Disease Prevention Programme

† Research Biochemist, Sydney Coronary Heart Disease Prevention Programme, and Scientific Officer, Department of Medicine, St. Vincent's Hospital, Sydney

MTPPRESS LIMITED *International Medical Publishers*

Lipids:
A Clinicians' Guide

Published in UK, Europe and Middle East
by MTP Press Limited
Falcon House
Lancaster
England

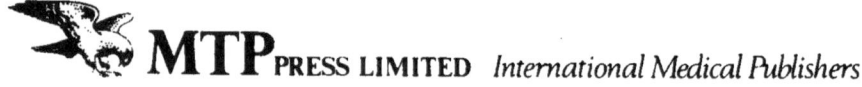 **MTP**PRESS LIMITED *International Medical Publishers*

ISBN 978-0-85200-511-8   ISBN 978-94-010-9464-1 (eBook)
DOI 10.1007/978-94-010-9464-1

Foreword

Coronary heart disease is the principal cause of death in all Western countries. Abnormalities in the serum lipids are one of the major risk factors widely recognised as leading to this epidemic of heart disease. These abnormalities occur very commonly in the general community and in general practice, and practitioners are prevailed upon daily to provide specific advice about diet and cholesterol and to interpret chemical estimations.

This is a very emotive area of medicine, one where often the patients most active in seeking advice have the least to gain. On the other hand, there may be young people carrying a severe coronary risk, knowingly or not, who prefer to avoid risk factor intervention. There are strong vested interests in the commercial world who would prefer to overlook any therapeutic value of dietary modification for selected individuals, and others who see great merit in a particular diet. The pharmaceutical industry has a vested interest in the cholesterol story as well. The individual doctor needs to decide for himself whether the cholesterol issue requires action or not, and for this he needs access to up to date and relevant data. This is one of the purposes of this book.

The use of lipid-lowering therapy is usually quite a straightforward exercise for any medical practitioner, once the decision has been taken to initiate it. This book attempts to give the clinician, be he general practitioner, cardiologist, physician or senior medical student, the background information on the subject of lipids, so that he may make a rational decision whether or not to initiate therapy. The book follows a logical sequence of development: key areas of biochemistry are discussed briefly, followed by an exposition of the important clinical implications of abnormal lipid values. Passing reference is made to other important risk factors, but their modification is not discussed in any detail. The evidence to justify risk factor intervention and the treatment of hyperlipidaemia is presented in detail. If the reader is convinced that a case for treatment exists, in general or in particular, then he will find details of diagnosis and management in the final two chapters.

This is not intended to be an exhaustive textbook on the subject of lipids. Several rare or unusual problems have received scant mention or have been omitted, but there are a number of textbooks providing such coverage. It is hoped that this book will function as a practical guide, providing material of use to all branches of the medical profession. The authors do not see any fundamental difference in the role of specialist or general practitioner in regard to diagnosis and management of lipid abnormality. It is acknowledged that in certain countries the availability of key drugs might prevent general practitioners from initiating certain therapy.

The cholesterol field is in turmoil on the subject of units, milligrams or millimoles. All the basic epidemiological research has been published in mg units and all American work continues in this way. More recent non-American work is reported in SI units. The practitioner these days really needs to be conversant with both systems, although it is preferable that SI units only be used. To be consistent with these aims, the authors have presented original results in the units in which they were first published. At times equivalent values have also been provided. For practical purposes, 1 mmol/litre cholesterol is approximately equivalent to 39mg/100ml, while 1 mmol/litre triglyceride is approximately equivalent to 89mg/100ml.

Acknowledgements

The authors wish to acknowledge the dedicated work of all the technical and nursing staff associated with the Lipid Laboratory at St. Vincent's Hospital. The expert secretarial assistance of Miss Suellen Maunder is also gratefully acknowledged.

Contents

Chapter I

Plasma Lipids and Lipoproteins

Lipids are a heterogeneous group of compounds which are grouped together by virtue of their solubility in organic solvents and insolubility in aqueous media. The blood lipids comprise free and esterified cholesterol, triglycerides, phospholipids and free fatty acids. Free cholesterol is the form of the sterol important functionally for membrane formation, hormone and bile acid synthesis, whereas cholesterol ester predominates in transport and storage forms of the sterol.

Plasma lipoproteins are an evolutionary adaptation facilitating the transport of the water insoluble blood lipids in an aqueous medium — the blood plasma or serum. Current concepts of lipoprotein structure strongly support a general model in which the more hydrophobic lipids (triglyceride and cholesterol ester) are surrounded by phospholipids, free cholesterol, and protein in an as yet undefined array [1]. Free fatty acids are not bound to plasma lipoproteins to any appreciable degree, but rather are transported with plasma albumin.

1. Lipoprotein Classification and Composition

The major lipoproteins are shown in table I. These lipoprotein classes have been defined by two operational criteria, ultracentrifugal flotation and electrophoretic mobility. The ultracentrifugal terminology: chylomicrons, VLDL, LDL, HDL (i.e. very low, low and high density lipoproteins) will be used here exclusively.

Each lipoprotein class is discrete with respect to the type and amount of lipid and protein. Chylomicrons and VLDL are dynamic molecules whose principal role is the transport of energy in the form of triglyceride to peripheral tissues. In contrast, LDL and HDL are the major cholesterol transporting lipoproteins, the former apparently involved in the transfer of cholesterol to the tissues and the latter important in the

Table I. Composition and classification of the major human plasma lipoproteins (weight percent)

Feature	Chylo-microns	VLDL	LDL[1]	HDL
Density (g/ml)	< 1.006	< 1.006	1.006-1.063	1.063-1.21
Electrophoretic mobility	Origin	Pre*beta*	*beta*	*alpha*
Triglyceride	85-90	50-55	6-10	3-6
Cholesterol ester	3-4	14-16	35-45	12-18
Unesterified cholesterol	2-3	6-8	8-12	2-4
Phospholipid	6-8	16-20	20-25	25-30
Protein	1-2	8-10	18-22	47-52

1 LDL is frequently separated into 2 density classes, IDL, 1.006-1.019g/ml and LDL$_2$, 1.019-1.063g/ml as discussed in section 1.3.

removal of cholesterol from peripheral sites to sites of degradation and excretion. Traditionally, emphasis has been placed on the lipid content of these lipoproteins but, during the past 15 years, the functional and structural significance of the specific lipid binding proteins of the lipoproteins, the apoproteins, has been increasingly appreciated.

The A B C nomenclature for the apolipoproteins, first suggested by Alaupovic [2], has been used in table II, which sets out the distribution among the lipoproteins of the major apoproteins characterised thus far. These apoproteins appear to have both structural and catalytic functions. The C peptides, for example, are transferred from HDL to chylomicrons and VLDL in a process facilitating the degradation of the latter lipoproteins [3]. Apo A-I performs an important functional role in the metabolism of HDL cholesterol ester. Apo D may serve to catalyse cholesterol ester exchange from HDL to VLDL [4]. In contrast, apo B, the major apoprotein of LDL, may serve a primarily structural role in maintaining the integrity of chylomicrons and VLDL during their transformation to LDL, and apo A-II may be an integral structural component of HDL. Potential functional roles for apo B and apo E are suggested in section 4.2, where their interactions with a specific cell surface receptor mediating lipoprotein catabolism are discussed.

1.1 Chylomicrons

Chylomicron is the term originally used in 1920 to describe the microscopically visible particles appearing in the plasma after a fatty meal [5]. Subsequently, chylomicrons have been characterised as triglyceride-rich particles secreted by the intestine, the major transport form of dietary fat. During digestion, dietary fat is emulsified and hydrolysed in the lumen of the duodenum by the combined actions of pancreatic lipase and biliary secretions. Fatty acids of fewer than 10 carbon units are transported via the portal circulation directly to the liver. Other degradation products, largely monoglycerides and free fatty acids of greater than 10 carbon units, enter the intestinal mucosal cell and serve as precursors in triglyceride synthesis. The re-synthesised triglyceride is combined with cholesterol and small amounts of phospholipid and specific apoproteins (apo B, apo A-I, apo C and apo E) to form the chylomicron molecule [6]. The importance of lipoprotein protein synthesis for chylomicron formation is emphasised by the inherited syndrome of abetalipoproteinaemia, characterised by fat malabsorption due to the inability to synthesise apo B and to form chylomicrons.

The chylomicron molecules reach the systemic circulation via the thoracic lymph. Once in the general circulation, they are modified in several ways. Primary modification involves the transfer from HDL of the C peptides and of apo E. This enriches the chylomicron with apo C-II, the co-factor needed for enzymatic removal of triglyceride. Subsequent modification involves interaction with adipose and other peripheral tissues leading to loss of lipid and protein in a sequence to be discussed later (section 4.1). The high concentration of triglyceride in the blood during the absorptive phase of digestion largely reflects chylomicron input.

1.2 Very Low Density Lipoproteins

VLDL share many metabolic and physical properties with chylomicrons. They serve a transport function for triglyceride and though generally of smaller diameter (280-750A), may overlap chylomicrons in the lower density ranges. A primary distinction between VLDL and chylomicrons is in the origin of the transported tri-

Table II. Apoprotein composition of human plasma lipoproteins

Lipoprotein class	Chylomicron	VLDL	LDL	HDL
Major apoproteins	A-I, A-II B C-I, C-II, C-III E	B C-I, C-II, C-III E	B	A-I, A-II
Minor and trace apoproteins		A-I, A-II	C-I, C-II, C-III	C-I, C-II, C-III D E

glyceride. In contrast to the transport of dietary fat, VLDL transport triglycerides derived from endogenous sources. The liver is the principal source of VLDL but, in the post-absorptive and fasting states, the intestine secretes a VLDL-sized particle containing triglyceride synthesised in the intestinal mucosa.

It is not known with certainty whether these intestinal VLDL are more closely related to chylomicrons or to hepatic VLDL, but the apoprotein composition suggests that chylomicrons and intestinal VLDL represent a class of lipoproteins which should be distinguished from hepatic VLDL [6-8]. Plasma VLDL contain approximately 8 to 10% protein, the principal apoproteins being apo B, apo C, and apo E [9].

1.3 Low Density Lipoproteins

In contrast to the major role played by chylomicrons and VLDL in the transport of triglyceride, the low density and high density lipoproteins are the major cholesterol transporting lipoproteins.

LDL contain, by weight, 80% lipid and 20% protein. Consistent with this increased protein content, LDL are smaller (210-250A) and are of higher flotation density (1.006-1.063g/ml) than VLDL and chylomicrons. 60% of LDL lipid is cholesterol and this represents approximately 70% of the total plasma cholesterol. LDL is the major form of circulating cholesterol. Apo B is the major apoprotein of normal LDL and represents 90 to 95% of the total plasma apo B. Experimental evidence suggests that the LDL apo B in normal man is derived almost entirely from VLDL apo B in plasma [10]. LDL is frequently separated into two classes, IDL and LDL_2, on the basis of flotation density. The lower density fraction, IDL (d = 1.006 - 1.019g/ml) is more lipid-rich than LDL_2 (d = 1.019 - 1.063g/ml) and probably represents an intermediate in VLDL catabolism. Thus, a comparison of IDL with LDL_2 demonstrates the gradual disappearance of triglyceride and of apoproteins more characteristic of VLDL (apo C and apo E), and an enrichment with apo B and cholesterol ester.

1.4 High Density Lipoproteins

The HDL molecule contains approximately 50% protein and 50% lipid. HDL are the smallest lipoproteins (90-120A) and float at the highest density (1.063-1.21g/ml) of any of the lipoprotein molecules. The quantitatively most important HDL lipid is phospholipid, although HDL cholesterol is of particular interest. The major phospholipid species is phosphatidylcholine (also known as lecithin), accounting for 70 to 80% of the total phospholipid. It has an important functional role in plasma cholesterol esterification, as a reactant in the enzymatic reaction catalysed by lecithin cholesterol acyl transferase (LCAT) [section 3.4].

HDL has been separated into two subclasses, HDL_2 (1.063-1.125g/ml) and HDL_3 (1.125-1.21g/ml). HDL levels have been shown to vary inversely with cardiovascular disease risk and most of this variation appears to be derived from changes in HDL_2 [11]. Females, for example, have higher HDL_2 levels than males but similar amounts of HDL_3. The major apoproteins of HDL are apo A-I and apo A-II, the former predominating. Apo A-I has been shown to be an activator of the LCAT reaction. In addition to these two proteins, HDL provides a reservoir of apo C peptides and contains apo D, apo E, and perhaps other trace apoproteins [12].

In addition to the major lipoprotein classes, two further lipoproteins deserve separate comment.

1.5 Lp(a) Lipoprotein

Similarities in lipid composition, concentration and density (1.05-1.10g/ml) between Lp(a) and LDL prevented clear discrimination of these two lipoproteins until immunological tests demonstrated the uniqueness of their protein moieties. 65% of Lp(a) protein is apo B, but another 15% is albumin and the remainder is an apoprotein unique to Lp(a), called apo Lp(a). Despite a high prevalence in the community [13], the functional significance is uncertain.

1.6 Lp-X Lipoprotein

Another lipoprotein with flotation density similar to that of LDL is Lp-X, although the lipid and protein compositions are quite different. This abnormal lipoprotein is characterised by an unusually high proportion of phospholipid and unesterified cholesterol, and by a low protein content consisting of apo B, apo C and albumin. It is found most characteristically in plasma of patients with biliary obstruction. The usual 'disc-like' structure of Lp-X as viewed with the electron microscope is similar to a lipoprotein of low density seen in LCAT deficiency. This suggests that Lp-X may arise as a result of incomplete modification of nascent HDL by LCAT.

2. Lipoprotein Metabolism

Plasma lipid concentrations are static indices of lipoprotein metabolism which are valuable in assessing cardiovascular risk. A complete understanding of factors determining blood lipid levels is the key to understanding the pathophysiology of hyperlipidaemia. These factors include anabolic processes such as absorption and synthesis, and catabolic processes such as mobilisation, degradation and excretion.

2.1 Absorption: Role of Dietary Triglyceride in the Regulation of Plasma Lipoprotein Levels

In the absorptive state, plasma triglyceride levels reflect chylomicron and intestinal VLDL synthesis and secretion, and respond accordingly to changes in both the amount and type of dietary fat. Dietary triglyceride is nearly completely absorbed and results in a postprandial rise in plasma triglyceride which peaks 3 to 5 hours after a meal. This peak is greater after a high fat than after a low fat meal. Chylomicron triglyceride is normally rapidly metabolised within 15 minutes of reaching the circulation, explaining why plasma triglyceride levels fluctuate with meal patterns. The measurement of triglyceride after a 12 to 14 hour overnight fast has the advantage of avoiding these fluctuations. This approach ignores postprandial tides of chylomicron triglyceride, which might better reflect arterial exposure to potentially atherogenic lipoproteins [14], but measurement of fasting triglyceride is recommended because of the difficulty of interpreting a single casual triglyceride determination.

A total quantity of dietary fat between 22 and 40 % of total calories does not appear to influence the plasma cholesterol level in man [15]. Extremely low levels of dietary fat, however, may reduce cholesterol levels by interference with cholesterol absorption, possibly because gallbladder contraction does not occur. This leads to a lack of biliary constituents which are needed for the micellar solubilisation of cholesterol.

The quality of dietary fat as opposed to quantity may exert an effect on blood levels of both triglyceride and cholesterol. It was recognised many years ago that the exchange of polyunsaturated fat for saturated fat in the diet could decrease plasma cholesterol levels in normal and hypercholesterolaemic individuals [16]. The mechanism of this cholesterol-lowering action is still poorly understood [17].

In addition to the cholesterol-lowering effect of polyunsaturated fats, a concomitant triglyceride-lowering effect has been documented [18]. In those individuals showing decrements in both plasma cholesterol and triglyceride with polyunsaturated fats, the cholesterol changes may be linked to changes in intestinal lipoprotein triglyceride degradation. Specifically, changes in fatty acid composition of chylomicrons and of intestinal VLDL triglycerides have been proposed to alter lipoprotein structure and subsequent metabolism [19]. Regardless of the aetiology, exchange of polyunsaturated fat for saturated in the diet has important therapeutic potential for hyperlipidaemic individuals.

2.2 Role of Dietary Cholesterol in Regulation of Plasma Lipids

In contrast to the diurnal fluctuation in plasma triglyceride levels, plasma cholesterol levels are relatively stable and do not reflect the chylomicron tide. This is consistent with the quantitatively small contribution made by chylomicrons and

VLDL to total plasma cholesterol transport (table I). Nevertheless, dietary cholesterol is absorbed in the chylomicron molecule and may have sustained effects on plasma cholesterol levels through regulation of endogenous cholesterol synthesis [20].

Dietary cholesterol consists of both free and esterified cholesterol. In the proximal small intestine, exogenous cholesterol is mixed with endogenous cholesterol from bile and sloughed cells, while cholesterol ester is hydrolysed by the action of pancreatic cholesterol esterase. The free cholesterol is absorbed with dietary triglyceride as a mixed micelle. In the intestinal mucosa approximately half of the free cholesterol is re-esterified with fatty acids from endogenous and exogenous sources and packaged into chylomicron molecules. Thus, chylomicron cholesterol esters reflect the fatty acid composition of the diet [21]. In contrast to dietary triglyceride, only 30 to 50% of dietary cholesterol is absorbed. The percentage absorption appears to be independent of cholesterol intake over a wide range of dietary cholesterol (fig. 1). It is clear that the more cholesterol one eats the more one absorbs. An important question then is 'what effect does this absorbed cholesterol have on long term plasma cholesterol levels?'

The relationship between dietary cholesterol intake and chronic plasma cholesterol concentration has been the subject of controversy for many years [22,23]. It is not disputed that in experimental animals cholesterol enriched diets readily elevate plasma cholesterol to pathological levels associated with atheroma development [24].

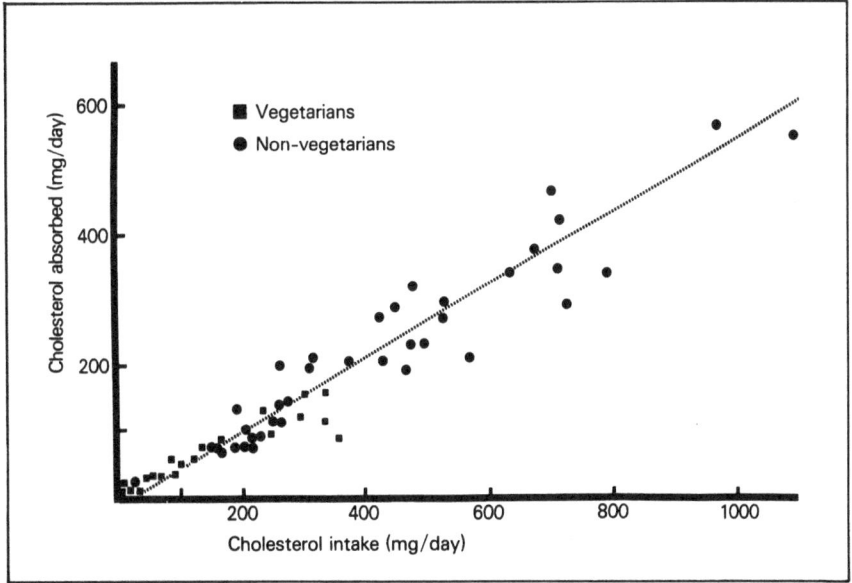

Fig. 1. The relationship between dietary cholesterol intake and cholesterol absorption over a wide range of cholesterol intakes in vegetarians and non-vegetarians.

The validity of extrapolating these data to a causal relationship in man is more doubtful. Controlled studies have demonstrated quite clearly that dietary cholesterol, in the range usually consumed in the diet of Western man, *will elevate plasma choles- terol levels above a baseline value established on a very low or cholesterol-free diet.* Glueck and Connor [22] have recently reviewed this evidence. Furthermore, popula- tions consuming diets markedly lower in cholesterol content than conventional Western diets have correspondingly lower plasma cholesterol levels. A positive rela- tionship between dietary cholesterol and plasma cholesterol levels has also been dem- onstrated in men of Japanese ancestry living in Japan, Hawaii, and California who consumed diets varying widely in cholesterol content [25].

Within a given community, however, a relationship in the individual subject bet- ween cholesterol intake and plasma cholesterol level is rarely demonstrable. This lack of correlation does not appear to be attributable to variations in cholesterol absorption [26]. The reasons underlying the lack of association are complex, but may be due in part to interactions with other dietary components such as dietary triglyceride and carbohydrate [27]. Also, limitations inherent in methods of obtaining precise dietary information may obscure correlations between dietary and biochemical parameters in individuals presenting small differences.

Perhaps most importantly, genetic factors contribute a great deal of interin- dividual variability in the 'baseline' value upon which the effects of dietary and other variables are superimposed [28]. Thus environmental factors including diet probably do modulate plasma cholesterol levels but within the bounds set by genetic determi- nants. A new aspect of this question has recently been introduced: studies have shown that regardless of whether total plasma cholesterol levels are influenced, inges- tion of cholesterol may result in the accumulation of a lipoprotein molecule with pathological potential in terms of altering cellular cholesterol metabolism [29].

3. Hepatic Lipoprotein Synthesis

In addition to the contribution made to plasma lipids by intestinal lipoproteins, the anabolic phase of lipoprotein metabolism involves synthesis and secretion of endogenous lipoproteins by the liver.

3.1 VLDL Synthesis

By analogy with chylomicron formation, the major stimulus to hepatic VLDL synthesis is the demand for triglyceride transport. In the intestine this demand is created by influx of dietary fat, but in the liver the stimulus is the availability of pre- cursors for endogenous triglyceride synthesis. As shown in figure 2, these precursors are non-esterified or free fatty acids and activated glycerol, (α-glycerophosphate). Free fatty acids are the principal stimulus to triglyceride synthesis and arise from three sources, the quantitative significance of which varies with the metabolic state. In the absorptive state, glucose and residual chylomicron triglyceride fatty acids serve as fatty acid precursors, while in the post-absorptive state free fatty acids mobilised from adipose tissue predominate.

After the postprandial rise in chylomicron triglyceride, a secondary rise in triglyceride concentration occurs 4 to 6 hours after a meal. This represents predominantly hepatic VLDL triglyceride synthesised from glucose and chylomicron triglyceride not hydrolysed in peripheral tissue. The relative contributions of glucose and dietary fat vary with diet composition. Institution of a high carbohydrate diet may lead to a phenomenon known as carbohydrate-induced hypertriglyceridaemia. With high dietary carbohydrate, glucose influx into the hepatocyte is in excess of both energy demands and of glycogen storage capacity. This results in shunting of acetyl CoA into fatty acid synthesis and of dihydroxy-acetone phosphate into activated glycerol (fig. 2). Thus the enzymatic machinery is tuned for triglyceride synthesis. This phenomenon may not persist in normal individuals but others may be unusually susceptible to carbohydrate induction of VLDL synthesis. This is the basis for reduction of dietary carbohydrate in the treatment of hypertriglyceridaemia, but this approach is unsuccessful if the hypertriglyceridaemia is due to other causes of overproduction or to a clearance defect. Other hypertriglyceridaemic states due to enhanced hepatic VLDL triglyceride synthesis include alcoholism [30] and oestrogen therapy [31].

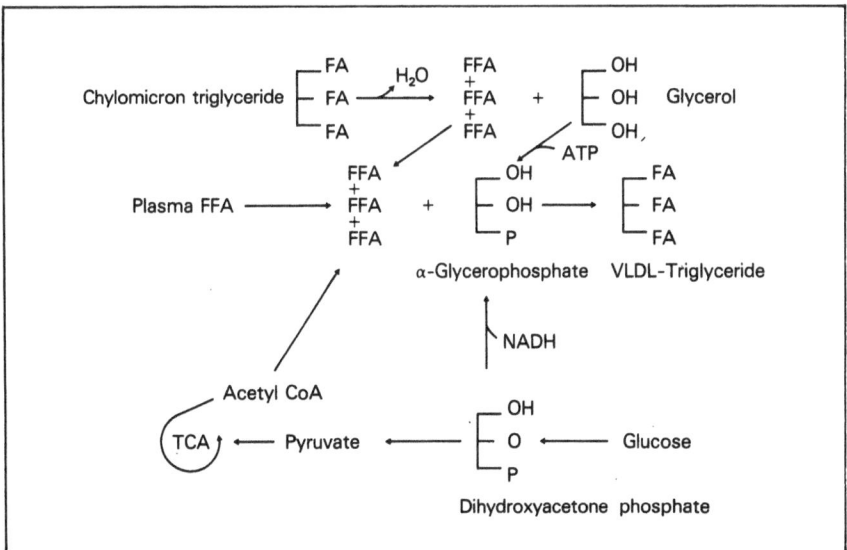

Fig. 2. Schematic representation of VLDL triglyceride synthesis (FFA, free fatty acids).

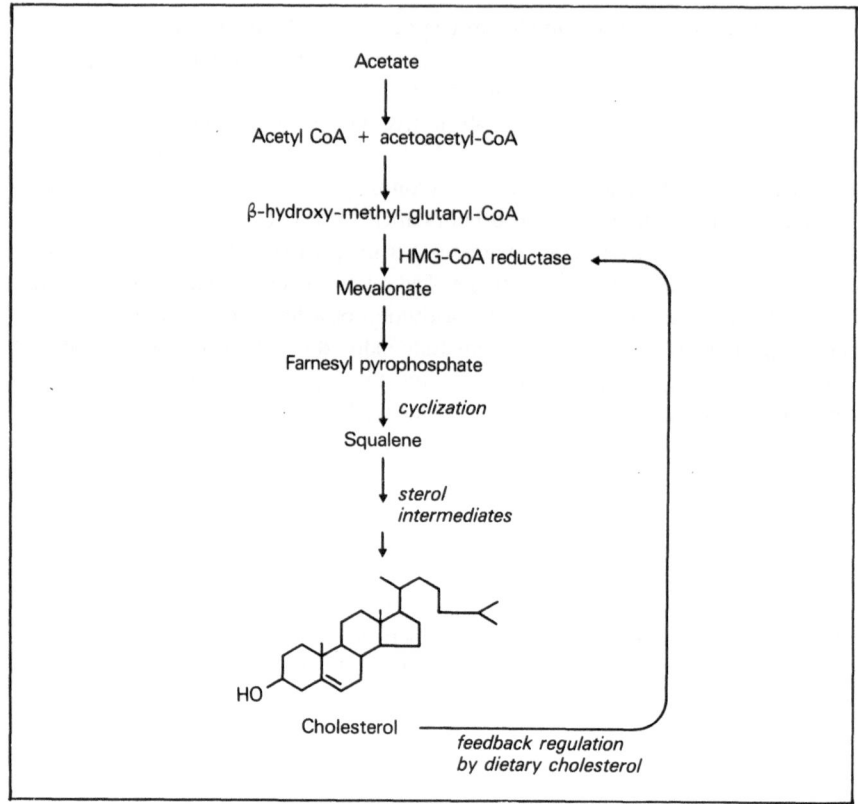

Fig. 3. The major steps in cholesterol biosynthesis from acetate.

3.2 Hepatic Cholesterol Synthesis

Though the primary stimulus to VLDL synthesis is triglyceride transport, cholesterol, phospholipid and protein are necessary for lipoprotein synthesis and secretion. Cholesterol synthesis in particular has been shown to be related to the demand for triglyceride transport [32]. All tissues of the body are capable of cholesterol synthesis but the liver and intestine are the major sources of endogenous cholesterol destined for transport.

The major steps in cholesterol biosynthesis from acetate are outlined in figure 3. The rate limiting enzyme is HMG-CoA reductase catalysing the reduction of B-hydroxy-methyl-glutaryl-CoA to form mevalonic acid. This enzyme in the liver is regulated by dietary cholesterol and by the enterohepatic circulation of bile salts. Specifically, the rate of hepatic cholesterol synthesis is inversely related to hepatic cholesterol uptake from chylomicrons and intestinal VLDL [20]. Procedures interfering with bile acid availability also enhance cholesterol synthesis via HMG-CoA reductase, but this effect may be secondary to an effect on cholesterol metabolism [33]. Ion exchange resins such as cholestyramine bind bile acids, increase conversion of cholesterol to bile acid and hence increase cholesterol synthesis. The degree of cholesterol lowering effected by cholestyramine is dependent upon the extent to which steroid excretion is increased relative to this increase in hepatic cholesterogenesis.

It might be inferred from this relation between dietary cholesterol and cholesterol synthesis that variations in dietary cholesterol can easily be monitored and cholesterol pools adjusted accordingly. Dietary cholesterol does however modify individual cholesterol levels and this suggests a more complex relationship, perhaps relating to cholesterol synthesis by extra-hepatic tissues which are not directly responsive to chylomicron cholesterol.

Hepatic biosynthesis of triglyceride, cholesterol and phospholipid occurs in the smooth endoplasmic reticulum. These lipid components contribute to the lipoprotein core and the surface coat respectively but, as in the intestine, apoprotein incorporation is essential prior to secretion. Apo B in particular is necessary for hepatic VLDL production as demonstrated by the complete absence of plasma VLDL and accumulation of hepatic lipids in abetalipoproteinaemia [34]. In addition to apo B, apo C and apo E appear to be components of nascent hepatic VLDL [35]. The products of lipid and protein biosynthesis are packaged for release in the hepatic Golgi apparatus, where addition of a carbohydrate moiety may be an important preliminary event to secretion via the space of Disse.

3.3 LDL Synthesis

All available evidence points to the formation of LDL in man as a catabolic by-product of VLDL and perhaps chylomicron metabolism, and this is discussed in section 4.1. It has been suggested that a VLDL-independent source of plasma LDL exists in homozygous familial hypercholesterolaemia, a syndrome which is characterised by an abnormally high rate of LDL synthesis [36]. This may be an exaggeration of a normally minor synthetic pathway.

3.4 HDL Synthesis

Nascent HDL molecules are synthesised in intestinal mucosal cells [37] and in hepatocytes [38] by a process analogous to that of VLDL and chylomicron synthesis. This involves microsomal lipid and protein synthesis, followed by Golgi packaging and secretion. Factors regulating HDL synthesis have not yet been defined. Ethanol is one factor which appears to elevate HDL levels [39], perhaps by increasing hepatic HDL synthesis. During the synthetic process, phospholipid and free cholesterol are

combined with specific apoproteins to form disc-like structures which undergo extensive compositional and structural modifications after secretion. The most important
of these modifications is the esterification of free cholesterol to form cholesterol ester
by an enzymatic reaction catalysed by LCAT (fig. 4). In man this is the major source
of plasma cholesterol esters. Individuals with LCAT deficiency have an accumulation
of these cholesterol ester deficient particles in plasma [40]. This suggests that the
cholesterol ester formed in the LCAT reaction allows the expansion of the disc-like
structures to form spheres characteristic of normal plasma HDL. Cholesterol ester
thus formed may be transferred to VLDL during catabolism [41].

   The apoprotein profile of nascent HDL is modified concomitantly with changes
in lipid content. Apo E is a major component of newly secreted HDL [35] relative to
apo A and apo C, while plasma HDL is characterised by a predominance of apo A
with minor contributions by apo C and apo E. The functional significance of this

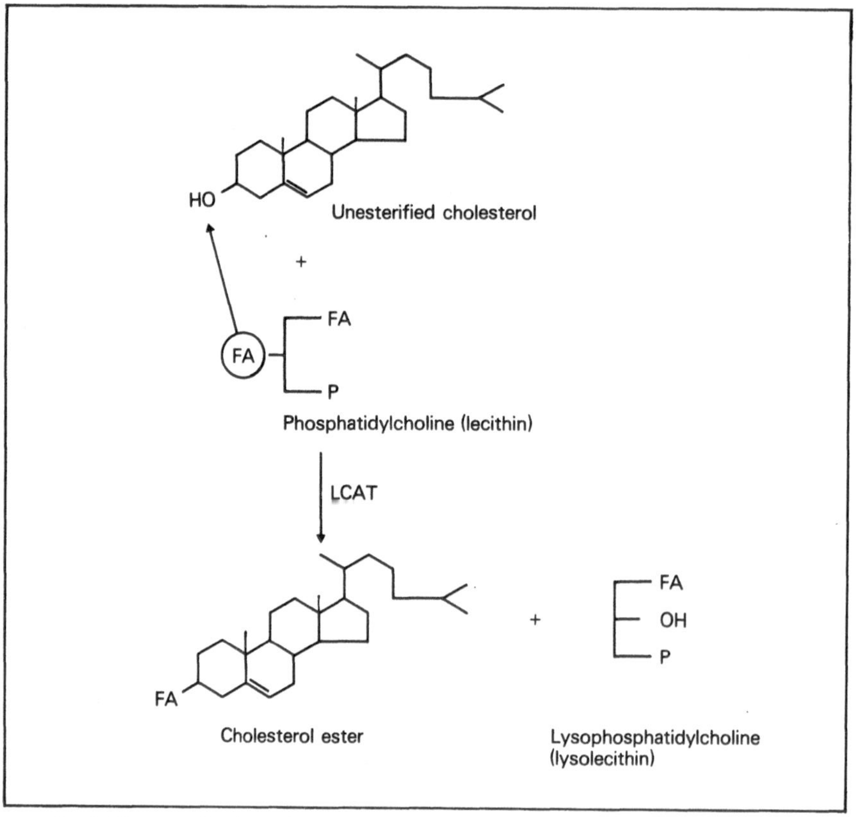

Fig. 4. The esterification of plasma cholesterol by the enzyme lecithin:cholesterol acyl
transferase (LCAT).

modification is not completely understood at present, but apo A-I is an activator of LCAT and its acquisition must facilitate the LCAT reaction.

4. Lipoprotein Catabolism

Plasma lipids are not the result of synthetic processes alone but reflect the effectiveness of opposing catabolic processes.

4.1 Chylomicron and VLDL Catabolism

The initiating step in the catabolism of both chylomicrons and VLDL is the acquisition of apo C-II from HDL. Apo C-II then catalyses lipoprotein triglyceride hydrolysis by the enzyme lipoprotein lipase. Lipoprotein lipase is localised on the luminal surface of the capillary endothelial cells of adipose tissue, muscle, lung, lactating mammary gland and in large arteries. Since the enzyme is released from endothelial cells into the circulation by heparin, plasma 'post heparin lipolytic activity' is frequently used as an index of lipoprotein-triglyceride hydrolysing capacity. Unfortunately this index is not completely reliable because of problems with assay standardisation and specificity. As shown in figure 5 lipoprotein lipase-catalysed hydrolysis results in progressive triglyceride depletion of the lipoprotein molecule through the IDL intermediate. This transformation involves maintenance of lipoprotein structure by simultaneous removal of phospholipid, unesterified cholesterol and apo C peptides from the lipoprotein surface to plasma HDL [42]. Reciprocal transfer of cholesterol ester from HDL may occur [4]. In man, it is by way of IDL or 'remnant' intermediates that VLDL is transformed into LDL [43], a process which focuses on VLDL metabolism as a determinant of LDL levels. During the transformation of VLDL to LDL, a constant amount of apo B is maintained per particle [44], indicating that apo B is a fundamental structural unit of chylomicrons, VLDL, intermediate and low density lipoproteins. Type III hyperlipidaemia is characterised by an accumulation of intermediate density particles, suggesting that this is a remnant disease caused by a defect in VLDL catabolism [45]. This LPL-mediated catabolism of VLDL and chylomicrons represents a critical step in lipoprotein metabolism and abnormalities may be manifested in several types of hyperlipidaemia (chapter IV, 2.1).

4.2 LDL Catabolism

The primary transport task of LDL appears to be the supply of cholesterol to peripheral tissues for membrane synthesis. Accordingly, LDL catabolism may be governed largely by the demand of cells for this cholesterol. Goldstein and Brown

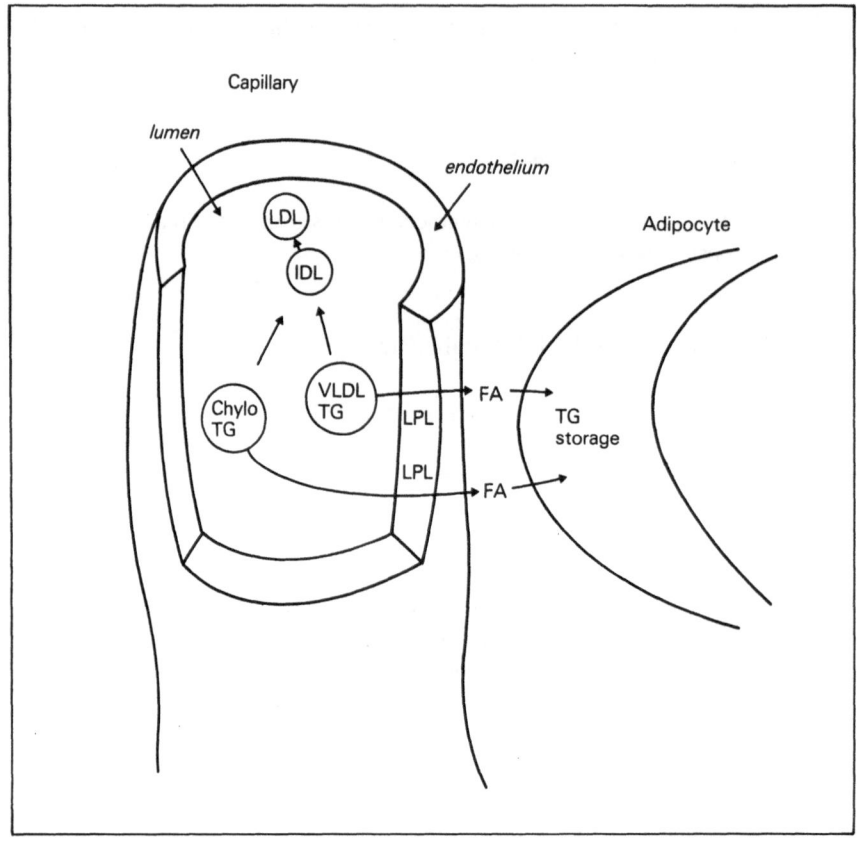

Fig. 5. Schematic representation of chylomicron and VLDL hydrolysis by lipoprotein lipase (LPL).

have contributed a great deal to the understanding of LDL catabolism through the recognition that in response to cholesterol availability cells synthesise a specific receptor which becomes translocated to the cell surface and binds LDL [46]. The steps of LDL catabolism as delineated by Goldstein and Brown are shown diagrammatically in figure 6.

These cell surface receptors bind LDL with high affinity and facilitate the internalisation of the whole LDL molecule. Lysosomal uptake is followed by hydrolysis of the LDL protein and cholesterol ester. The free cholesterol thus released may cross the lysosomal membrane and gain access to cellular compartments, where it is used for membrane synthesis and serves to regulate cholesterol synthesis via HMG-CoA reductase. This LDL internalisation also regulates synthesis of the LDL receptor itself. Cells grown in LDL-deficient serum have high rates of LDL binding and chol-

esterol synthesis and these are reduced after exposure to LDL. Excess cholesterol acti-
vates the enzyme acyl-CoA cholesterol acyl transferase (ACAT), leading to intracell-
ular cholesterol ester storage. Thus, the net result of LDL binding and internalisation
is the reciprocal inhibition and activation of enzymes synthesising and storing cellular
cholesterol and a reduction in the number of receptors available to bind LDL.

The pioneering work delineating this process was done with human fibroblasts
in tissue culture, but subsequent studies have verified the existence of similar path-
ways in lymphocytes [47], arterial smooth muscle cells [48] and non-confluent endothelial cells [49]. These findings suggest a potential role for peripheral tissues in LDL
binding and catabolism. Other studies in hepatectomised animals have provided additional evidence for the capacity of peripheral tissue to degrade LDL [50]. The potential
significance of this process for regulation of plasma cholesterol levels in man is
illustrated by patients with the homozygous form of familial hypercholesterolaemia.
These patients are deficient in LDL receptors and have excessive LDL production and
defective LDL catabolism [51], presumably due to an inability of tissues to bind, inter-
nalise, degrade and thus to regulate cholesterol synthesis. With the exception of this
receptor-deficient state of familial hypercholesterolaemia however, the role of the
LDL receptor in the final determination of plasma cholesterol levels is uncertain and
is probably only complementary to other regulatory processes. It has recently been
recognised that the specificity of the LDL receptor extends to lipoproteins containing
apo E as well as apo B. Lipoproteins of high density (1.063-1.125g/ml) are produced
by the feeding of cholesterol to both animals [52] and man [29] and this 'HDL$_c$' has an

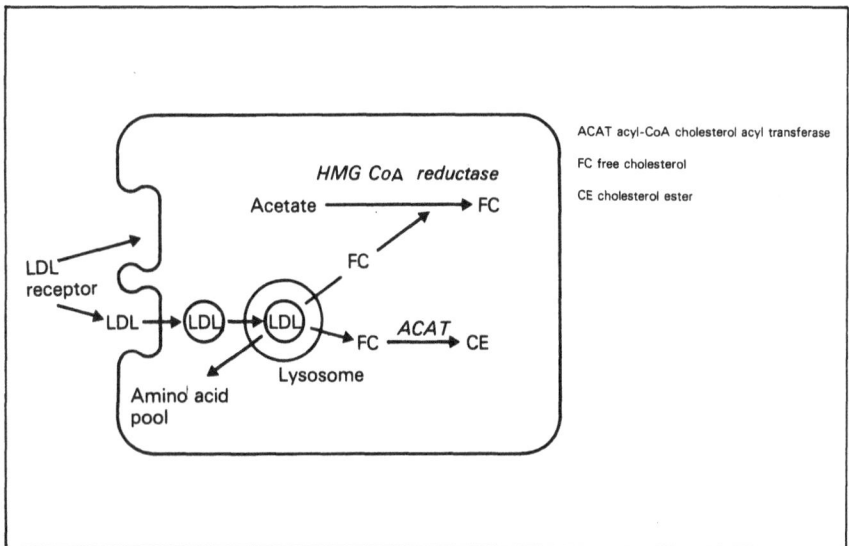

Fig. 6. Diagrammatic representation of LDL catabolism via specific cell surface receptors.

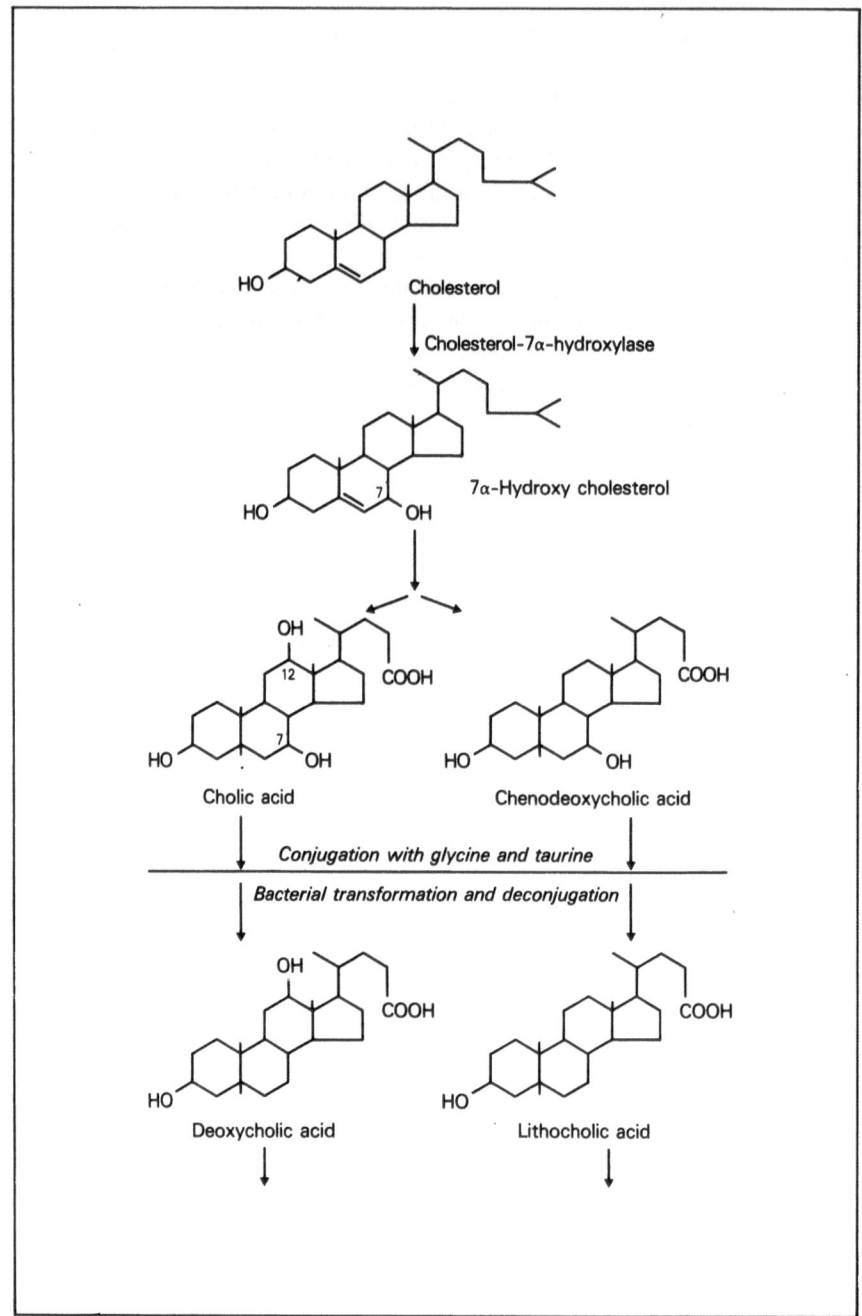

Fig. 7. Schematic representation of the transformation of cholesterol to bile acids.

increased content of apo E and enhanced capacity to interact with the LDL receptor [53].

In contrast, normal HDL may balance LDL transport by mediating cholesterol removal from peripheral sites to degradative and excretory sites. In tissue culture HDL has been shown to compete with LDL for receptor sites but to be internalised to a lesser degree and to enhance cholesterol efflux [54]. This role of HDL in 'reverse cholesterol transport' [48] may be the basis for the protection afforded by HDL against cardiovascular disease.

4.3 Cholesterol Excretion

The final step in the catabolism of lipoprotein lipids is cholesterol excretion and degradation via the hepato-biliary system in the form of neutral and acidic sterols. An estimate of faecal acidic and neutral sterol excretion may be used as a means of measuring changes in cholesterol metabolism since acidic and neutral sterol output reflect hepatic and peripheral cholesterol flux.

Faecal neutral sterols represent cholesterol and its bacterial degradation products from three sources: that which has been excreted by the liver, unabsorbed dietary cholesterol and cholesterol present in sloughed intestinal mucosal cells. Because of the heterogeneous nature of this cholesterol, radioisotopic labelling methods are required to distinguish cholesterol originating in lipoproteins (endogenous steroids) from that of gastrointestinal origin (exogenous steroid).

In addition to neutral sterol excretion, cholesterol removal is effected by the enzymatic transformation of cholesterol to bile acids. The major rate limiting step in hepatic bile acid synthesis is that catalysed by the enzyme cholesterol 7-alpha-hydroxylase, as illustrated in figure 7. Prior to excretion, the bile acids are conjugated with the amino acids glycine or taurine so that the final biliary products of cholesterol degradation are the primary bile acids, taurocholic, glycocholic, taurochenodeoxycholic and glycochenodeoxycholic acids. Glycine conjugates predominate in man. Further enzymatic deconjugation and bacterial transformation of these primary bile acids occur in the terminal ileum and colon. The final products of the cholesterol transformation to bile acids are the four unconjugated bile acids, cholic and chenodeoxycholic acids and their metabolites, deoxycholic and lithocholic acids.

As well as providing a pathway for cholesterol excretion, bile acids are critical for efficient fat absorption. Bile acids are secreted in the bile into the proximal intestine when gallbladder contraction occurs in response to dietary fat. Here they aid in the emulsification of dietary fat and activate pancreatic lipase (section 1.1). In the terminal ileum the bile acids are reabsorbed by active and passive transport, thus effecting considerable conservation of the bile acid pool (*circa* 95 %) via an enterohepatic circulation (fig. 8).

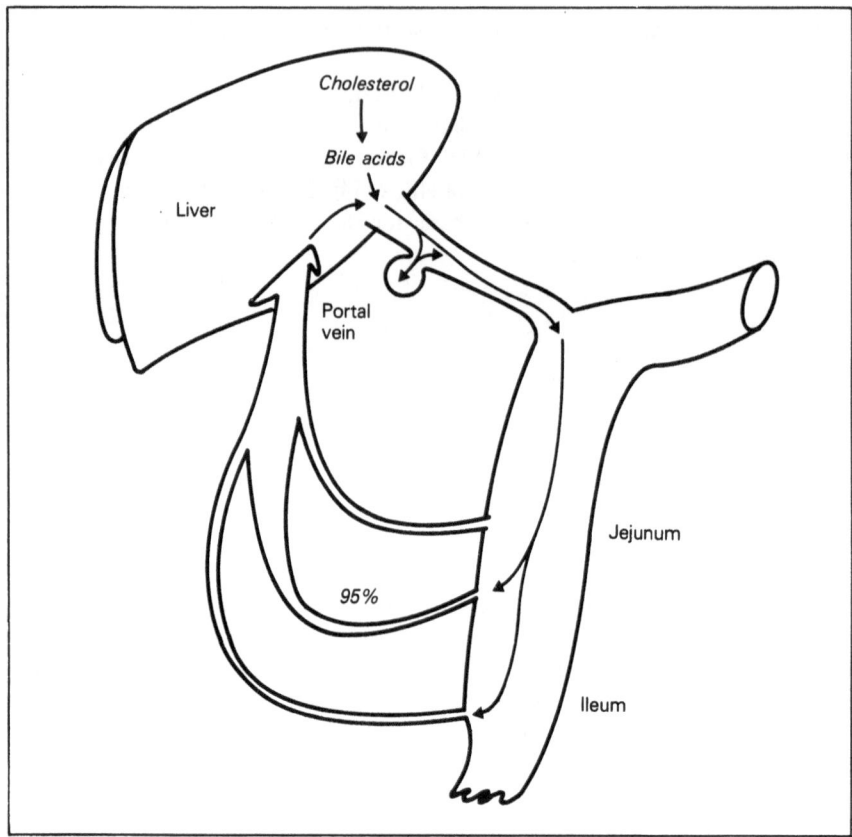

Fig. 8. The enterohepatic circulation of bile salts.

The concentration of bile acids returning to the liver by this enterohepatic circulation serves to regulate the activity of cholesterol 7-α-hydroxylase and thus the biosynthesis of bile acids from cholesterol. Resins such as cholestyramine sequester bile salts, interrupt the enterohepatic circulation, increase bile acid synthesis and consequently increase cholesterol excretion. This is the apparent mechanism of the plasma cholesterol-lowering action of cholestyramine.

The biosynthesis and metabolism of bile acids are also of significance in the aetiology of gallstone disease. The bile is the common vehicle for the excretion of cholesterol and bile acids serve the important function of solubilising cholesterol. Cholesterol gallstones, which account for about 70 % of all stones, are usually radioluscent and form when the capacity of the bile to solubilise cholesterol is exceeded [55]. The susceptibility to gallstone disease can be estimated by the degree of biliary cholesterol saturation (lithogenicity) as determined by biliary concentrations of cholesterol, bile salts and phospholipid [55]. Furthermore, treatments which change bile acid and/or cholesterol excretion affect cholesterol gallstone formation.

Dietary polyunsaturated fats, for example, have been associated with a slightly increased prevalence of cholelithiasis [56] which may reflect increased bile lithogenicity due to mobilisation of cholesterol into bile [57]. Treatment of hyperlipidaemia with clofibrate has been reported to result in a bile containing an increased concentration of cholesterol and a decreased concentration of bile salts [58] and has also been associated with an increased susceptibility to gallstone disease [59,60]. Feeding of chenodeoxycholic acid has been able to dissolve cholesterol gallstones in a proportion of cases and this effect may be due to feedback inhibition of cholesterol synthesis by chenodeoxycholate and associated reduction in biliary cholesterol [61]. Interestingly, this treatment may also decrease plasma triglyceride levels in hypertriglyceridaemic individuals, perhaps again by reducing cholesterol synthesis [62]. It is clear that cholesterol and bile acid synthesis and excretion are interrelated to the extent that primary alterations are difficult, if not impossible, to identify.

5. Pathogenesis of Atherosclerosis

An understanding of the risk factor relationship between hyperlipidaemia and cardiovascular disease should include consideration of the pathogenesis of atherosclerosis.

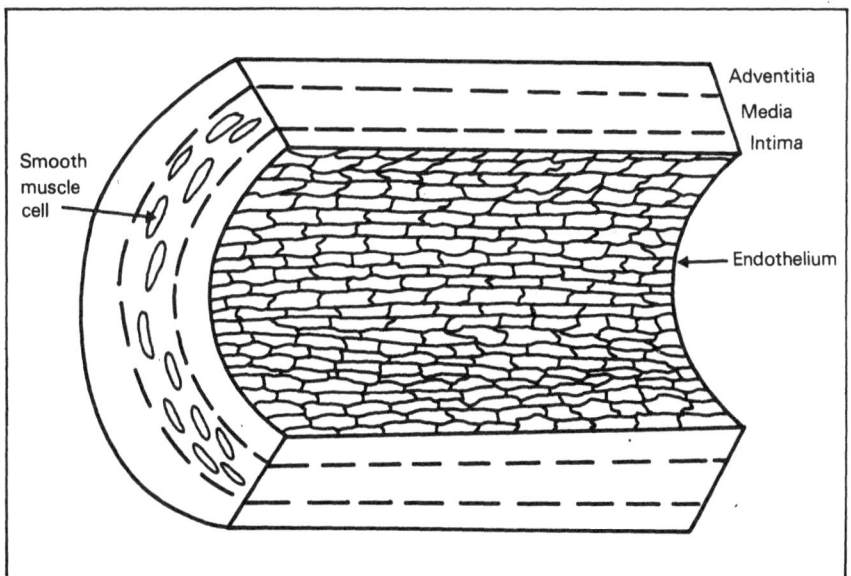

Fig. 9. Diagrammatic representation of the arterial wall.

The arterial wall is a complex structure comprising three morphologically distinct layers (fig. 9). In the healthy artery the intima is a region of smooth muscle cells interlaced with extracellular connective tissue. It is limited on the luminal side by a single layer of tightly apposed endothelial cells and on the other side by the internal elastic lamina. The media of the artery consists of circumferentially arranged smooth muscle cells surrounded by small amounts of collagen and elastin fibres. The adventitia or external coat is separated from the media by a poorly defined layer of elastic tissue and consists of fibroblasts, collagen and glycosoaminoglycans arranged in a loose array.

A developing atherosclerotic lesion goes through several stages. A focal thickening of the intima is a result of smooth muscle cell proliferation followed by accumulation of intra- and extracellular deposits of lipids, largely cholesterol. Advanced atherosclerosis is characterised by the development of a connective tissue cap encroaching upon the vessel lumen. A complicated lesion may develop as cells degenerate, blood elements enter and calcification occurs.

This sequence of events shows that lipid accumulation is a major and early step in the development of the atherosclerotic lesion. Although the normal arterial wall does actually synthesise cholesterol, evidence indicates that atheroma cholesterol is acquired from the plasma [63]. This view is reinforced by the finding of the plasma apo-lipoproteins, apo B and apo C in lesions [64].

That lipid is a component of the arterial lesion however does not identify it as a primary pathogenetic factor. In experimental studies a variety of stimuli including mechanical, biochemical and immunological factors have been shown to elicit lesion development. These stimuli share the property of providing an injury to the endothelial layer which normally serves as a permeability barrier to plasma components [65]. Regardless of the nature of the injury however, the proliferative response is accentuated by exposure to components of hyperlipidaemic plasma [66] and in experimental studies high plasma cholesterol levels are necessary for lesion development. LDL is avidly taken up by smooth muscle cells in culture and in addition is readily entrapped within the arterial wall by ionic interaction with connective tissue elements [67]. Thus, high levels of circulating LDL have proven potential for lesion perpetuation, if not initiation. The role of hyperlipidaemia in the initiation of atherosclerosis is less well defined although it has been proposed that the interaction of VLDL and chylomicrons with lipoprotein lipase during lipoprotein triglyceride hydrolysis may provoke focal arterial injury and allow lipid infiltration [14].

This view of the pathogenesis of atherosclerosis emphasises the multifactorial nature of cardiovascular disease risk; environmental factors such as high blood pressure or cigarette smoking may lead to endothelial injury and permeability changes, providing the opportunity for lipid infiltration and cell proliferation. Similarly, haemodynamic factors may contribute. Thus, any metabolic or environmental condition capable of arterial injury may, in the presence of hyperlipidaemia, lead to atherosclerosis and its complications.

Synopsis

Plasma cholesterol and triglyceride levels are the result of a dynamic equilibrium between anabolic and catabolic aspects of lipoprotein metabolism. Triglyceride levels reflect the extent to which chylomicron and VLDL input from the intestine and liver is balanced by lipoprotein lipase-catalysed triglyceride hydrolysis and subsequent utilisation. Factors enhancing lipoprotein production, or impairing removal, may alter the balance in favour of hypertriglyceridaemia.

Sources of cholesterol input are diet and endogenous synthesis, the latter predominating but under modulation by dietary input. Opposing forces, including cholesterol degradation by hepatic and extra-hepatic tissues, and excretion via the hepato-biliary system are equally important determinants of the steady-state level of plasma cholesterol.

LDL and HDL are the major cholesterol transporting lipoproteins. Plasma levels of these lipoproteins are affected by subtle changes in VLDL lipid and apoprotein composition. Hypercholesterolaemia consists of a heterogeneous group of disorders reflecting a primary alteration in either synthetic or degradative processes. The interdependence of these processes emphasises the difficulty in identifying the initiating factors in hyperlipidaemia.

References

1. Jackson, R.J.; Morrisett, J.D. and Gotto, Jr. A.M.: Lipoprotein structure and metabolism. Physiological Reviews 56: 259-316 (1976).
2. Alaupovic, P.; Lee, D.M. and McConathy, W.J.: Studies on the composition and structure of plasma lipoproteins. Distribution of lipoprotein families in major density classes of normal human plasma lipoproteins. Biochimica et Biophysica Acta 260: 689-707 (1072).
3. Havel, R.J.; Kane, J.P. and Kashyap, M.L.: Interchange of apolipoproteins between chylomicrons and high density lipoproteins during alimentary lipemia in man. Journal of Clinical Investigation 52: 32-38 (1973).
4. Chajek, T. and Fielding, C.J.: Isolation and characterization of human serum cholesteryl ester transfer protein. Proceedings of the National Academy of Sciences 75: 3445-3449 (1978).
5. Gage, S.H.: The free granules (chylomicrons) of the blood as shown by the dark field microscope. Cornell Veterinarian 10: 154-155 (1920).
6. Schonfeld, G.; Bell, E. and Alpers, D.H.: Intestinal lipoproteins during fat absorption. Journal of Clinical Investigation 62: 1539-1550 (1978).
7. Glickman, R.M. and Green, P.H.R.: The intestine as a source of apolipoprotein A-I. Proceedings of the National Academy of Sciences 74: 2569-2573 (1977).
8. Imaizumi, K.; Fainaru, M. and Havel, R.J.: Composition of proteins of mesenteric lymph chylomicrons in the rat and alterations produced upon exposure of chylomicrons to blood serum and serum proteins. Journal of Lipid Research 19: 712-722 (1978).
9. Kane, J.P.; Sata, T.; Hamilton, R.L. and Havel, R.J.: Apoprotein composition of very low density lipoproteins of human serum. Journal of Clinical Investigation 56: 1627-1634 (1975).

10. Sigurdsson, G.; Nicoll, A. and Lewis, B.: Conversion of very low density lipoprotein to low density lipoprotein. A metabolic study of apolipoprotein B kinetics in human subjects. Journal of Clinical Investigation 56: 1481-1490 (1975).

11. Anderson, D.W.: HDL Cholesterol: The variable component. Lancet 1: 819-820 (1978).

12. Shore, V.G.; Shore, B. and Lewis, S.B.: Isolation and characterization of two threonine-poor apolipoproteins of human plasma high density lipoproteins. Biochemistry 17: 2174-2178 (1978).

13. Albers, J.J. and Hazzard, W.R.: Immunochemical quantitation of human plasma Lp(a). Lipids 9: 15-26 (1974).

14. Zilversmit, D.B.: A proposal linking atherogenesis to the interaction of endothelial lipoprotein lipase with triglyceride-rich lipoproteins. Circulation Research 33: 633-638 (1973).

15. Hegsted, D.M.; McGandy, R.B.; Myers, M.L. and Stare, F.J.: Quantitative effects of dietary fat on serum cholesterol in man. American Journal of Clinical Nutrition 17: 281-295 (1965).

16. Kinsell, L.W.; Partridge, J.; Boling, L.; Margen, S. and Michaels, G.: Dietary modification of serum cholesterol and phospholipid levels. Journal of Clinical Endocrinology and Metabolism 12: 909-913 (1952).

17. Jackson, R.L.; Taunton, O.D.; Morrisett, J.D. and Gotto, Jr. A.M.: The role of dietary polyunsaturated fat in lowering blood cholesterol in man. Circulation Research 42: 447-453 (1978).

18. Grundy, S.M.: Effects of polyunsaturated fats on lipid metabolism in patients with hypertriglyceridemia. Journal of Clinical Investigation 55: 269-282 (1975).

19. Spritz, N. and Mishkel, M.A.: Effects of dietary fats on plasma lipids and lipoproteins: An hypothesis for lipid-lowering effect of unsaturated fatty acids. Journal of Clinical Investigation 48: 78-86 (1969).

20. Nervi, F.O. and Dietschy, J.M.: Ability of six different lipoprotein fractions to regulate the rate of hepatic cholesterogenesis. Journal of Biological Chemistry 250: 8704-8711 (1975).

21. Goodman, D.S.: Cholesterol ester metabolism. Physiological Reviews 45: 747-839 (1965).

22. Glueck, C.J. and Connor, W.E.: Diet — coronary heart disease relationships reconnoitered. American Journal of Clinical Nutrition 31: 727-737 (1978).

23. Reiser, R.: Oversimplification of diet: Coronary heart disease relationships and exaggerated diet recommendations. American Journal of Clinical Nutrition 31: 865-875 (1978).

24. Kritchevsky, D.: Experimental atherosclerosis in primates and other species. Annals of the New York Academy of Sciences 162: 80-87 (1969).

25. Kato, H.; Tillotson, J.; Nichaman, M.Z.; Rhoads, G.G. and Hamilton, H.: Epidemiologic studies of coronary heart disease and stroke in Japanese men living in Japan, Hawaii and California. American Journal of Epidemiology 97: 372-382 (1973).

26. Simons, L.A.; Gibson, J.C.; Paino, C.; Hosking, M.; Bullock, J. and Trim, J.: The influence of a wide range of absorbed cholesterol on plasma cholesterol levels in man. American Journal of Clinical Nutrition 31: 1334-1339 (1978).

27. McGandy, R.B.; Hegsted, D.M. and Stare, F.J.: Dietary fats, carbohydrates and atherosclerotic vascular disease. New England Journal of Medicine 277: 417-419, 469-471 (1967).

28. Hatch, F.T.: Interactions between nutrition and heredity in coronary heart disease. American Journal of Clinical Nutrition 27: 80-90 (1974).

29. Mahley, R.W.; Bersot, T.P.; Innerarity, T.L.; Lipson, A. and Margolis, S.: Alterations in human high-density lipoproteins, with or without increased plasma cholesterol, induced by diets high in cholesterol. Lancet 2: 807-809 (1978).

30. Lieber, C.S.: Effects of ethanol upon lipid metabolism. Lipids 9: 103-116 (1974).

31. Glueck, C.J.; Fallat, R.W. and Scheel, D.: Effects of estrogenic compounds on triglyceride kinetics. Metabolism 24: 537-545 (1975).

32. Sodhi, H.S. and Kudchodkar, B.J.: Synthesis of cholesterol in hypercholesterolemia and its relationship to plasma triglycerides. Metabolism 22: 895-912 (1973).

33. Nervi, F.O. and Dietschy, J.M.: The mechanisms of and the interrelationship between bile acid and

chylomicron-mediated regulation of hepatic cholesterol synthesis in the liver of the rat. Journal of Clinical Investigation 63: 895-909 (1978).

34. Parkin, J.S.; Partin, J.C.; Schubert, W.K. and McAdams, J.: Liver ultrastructure in abetalipoproteinemia: Evolution of micronodular cirrhosis. Gastroenterology 67: 107-118 (1974).

35. Marsh, J.B.: Apoproteins of the lipoproteins in a nonrecirculating perfusate of rat liver. Journal of Lipid Research 17: 85-90 (1976).

36. Soutar, A.K.; Myant, N.B. and Thompson, G.R.: Simultaneous measurement of apolipoprotein B turnover in very-low and low-density lipoproteins in familial hypercholesterolaemia. Atherosclerosis 28: 247-256 (1977).

37. Wu, A.L. and Windmueller, H.G.: Identification of circulating apolipoproteins synthesized by rat small intestine in vivo. Journal of Biological Chemistry 253: 2525-2531 (1978).

38. Hamilton, R.L.; Williams, M.C.; Fielding, C.J. and Havel, R.J.: Discoidal bilayer structure of nascent high density lipoproteins from perfused rat liver. Journal of Clinical Investigation 58: 667-680 (1976).

39. Castelli, W.P.; Doyle, J.T.; Gordon, T.; Halmes, C.G.; Hjortland, M.; Hulley, S.B.; Kagan, A. and Zukel, W.J.: Alcohol and blood lipids. The co-operative lipoprotein phenotyping study. Lancet 2: 153-155 (1977).

40. Forte, T.; Norum, K.R.; Glomset, J.A. and Nichols, A.V.: Plasma lipoproteins in familial lecithin: cholesterol acyl transferase deficiency: Structure of low and high density lipoproteins as revealed by electron microscopy. Journal of Clinical Investigation 50: 1141-1148 (1971).

41. Nichols, A.V. and Smith, L.: Effect of very low density lipoproteins on lipid transfer in incubated serum. Journal of Lipid Research 6: 206-210 (1965).

42. Patsch, J.R.; Gotto, Jr. A.M.; Olivecrona, T. and Eisenberg, S.: Formation of high density lipoprotein-like particles during lipolysis of very low density lipoproteins in vitro. Proceedings of the National Academy of Sciences 75: 4519-4523 (1978).

43. Eisenberg, S.; Bilheimer, D.W.; Levy, R.I. and Lindgren, F.T.: On the metabolic conversion of human plasma very low density lipoprotein to low density lipoprotein. Biochimica et Biophysica Acta 326: 361-377 (1973).

44. Mjos, O.D.; Faergeman, O.; Hamilton, R.L. and Havel, R.J.: Characterization of remnants produced during the metabolism of triglyceride-rich lipoproteins of blood plasma and intestinal lymph in the rat. Journal of Clinical Investigation 56: 603-615 (1975).

45. Havel, R.J. and Kane, J.P.: Primary dysbetalipoproteinemia: Predominance of a specific apoprotein species in triglyceride-rich lipoproteins. Proceedings of the National Academy of Sciences 70: 2015-2019 (1973).

46. Goldstein, J.L. and Brown, M.S.: The low density lipoprotein pathway and its relation to atherosclerosis. Annual Review of Biochemistry 46: 897-930 (1977).

47. Fogelman, A.M.; Edmond, J.; Seager, J. and Popjak, G.: Abnormal induction of 3-hydroxy-3-methylglutaryl Co enzyme A reductase in leukocytes from subjects with heterozygous familial hypercholesterolemia. Journal of Biological Chemistry 250: 2045-2055 (1975).

48. Weinstein, D.B.; Carew, T.E. and Steinberg, D.: Uptake and degradation of low density lipoprotein by swine arterial smooth muscle cells with inhibition of cholesterol biosynthesis. Biochimica et Biophysica Acta 424: 404-421 (1976).

49. Vlodavsky, I.; Fielding, P.E.; Fielding, C.J. and Gospodarowicz, D.: Role of contact inhibition in the regulation of receptor-mediated uptake of low density lipoprotein in cultured vascular endothelial cells. Proceedings of the National Academy of Sciences 75: 356-360 (1978).

50. Sniderman, A.D.; Carew, T.E.; Chandler, J.G. and Steinberg, D.: Paradoxical increase in rate of catabolism of LDL after hepatectomy. Science 183: 526-528 (1974).

51. Simons, L.A.; Reichl, D.; Myant, N.B. and Mancini, M.: The metabolism of the apoprotein of plasma low density lipoprotein in familial hyperbetalipoproteinaemia in the homozygous form. Atherosclerosis 21: 283-298 (1975).

52. Mahley, R.W.; Weisgraber, K.H. and Innerarity, T.: Canine lipoproteins and atherosclerosis. II. Characterization of the plasma lipoproteins associated with atherogenic and nonatherogenic hyperlipidemia. Circulation Research 35: 722-733 (1974).

53. Innerarity, T.L. and Mahley, R.W.: Enhanced binding by cultured human fibroblasts of apo-E-containing lipoproteins as compared with low density lipoproteins. Biochemistry 17: 1440-1446 (1978).

54. Miller, N.E.: Induction of low density lipoprotein receptor synthesis by high density lipoprotein in cultures of human skin fibroblasts. Biochimica et Biophysica Acta 529: 131-137 (1978).

55. Redinger, R.N. and Small, D.M.: Bile composition, bile salt metabolism, and gallstones. Archives of Internal Medicine 130: 618-630 (1972).

56. Sturdevant, R.A.L.; Pearce, M.L. and Dayton, S.: Increased prevalence of cholelithiasis in men ingesting a serum-cholesterol-lowering diet. The New England Journal of Medicine 288: 24-27 (1973).

57. Grundy, S.M.: Effects of polyunsaturated fats on lipid metabolism in patients with hypertriglyceridemia. Journal of Clinical Investigation 55: 269-282 (1975).

58. Pertsemlidis, D.; Panveliwalla, D. and Ahrens, E.H.: Effects of clofibrate and of an estrogen-progestin combination on fasting biliary lipids and cholic acid kinetics in man. Gastroenterology 66: 565-573 (1974).

59. Coronary Drug Project Research Group: Clofibrate and niacin in coronary heart disease. Journal of the American Medical Association 231: 360-381 (1975).

60. Committee of Principal Investigators: A co-operative trial in the primary prevention of ischaemic heart disease using clofibrate. British Heart Journal 40: 1069-1118 (1978).

61. Northfield, T.C.; LaRusso, N.F.; Hofmann, A.F. and Thistle, J.L.: Effect of chenodeoxycholic acid treatment in gallstone subjects. Gastroenterology 68: 12-17 (1975).

62. Miller, N.E. and Nestel, P.J.: Triglyceride lowering effect of chenodeoxycholic acid in patients with endogenous hypertriglyceridaemia. Lancet 2: 929-931 (1974).

63. Newman, H.A.I. and Zilversmit, D.B.: Quantitative aspects of cholesterol flux in rabbit atheromatous lesions. Journal of Biological Chemistry 237: 2078-2084 (1962).

64. Hoff, H.F.; Heideman, C.L.; Jackson, R.L. and Kim, H-S.: Localization patterns of plasma apolipoproteins in human atherosclerotic lesions. Circulation Research 37: 72-79 (1975).

65. Zilversmit, D.B. and Newman, H.A.I.: Does a metabolic barrier to circulatory cholesterol protect the arterial wall? Circulation 33: 7 (1966).

66. Fischer-Dzoga, K.; Fraser, R. and Wissler, R.W.: Stimulation of proliferation in stationary cultures of monkey and rabbit aortic smooth muscle cells. I. Effects of lipoprotein fractions of hyperlipemic serum and lymph. Experimental and Molecular Pathology 24: 346-359 (1976).

67. Srinivasan, S.R.; Dolan, P.; Radhakrishnamurthy, B.; Pargaonkar, P.S. and Berenson, G.S.: Lipoprotein acid mucopolysaccharide complexes of human atherosclerotic lesions. Biochimica et Biophysica Acta 388: 58-70 (1975).

Chapter II

Clinical Implications of Hyperlipidaemia

Hyperlipidaemia is usually a symptomless biochemical state which, if present for a sufficiently long time, may be associated with the development of atherosclerosis and its complications. Discussion of this important association constitutes the major portion of this chapter (section 1). Occasionally hyperlipidaemia may be associated with specific overt symptoms or signs directly attributable to the presence of hyperlipidaemia. Examples are the syndrome of hyperlipidaemia, abdominal pain and pancreatitis (section 2) and the cutaneous manifestations of hyperlipidaemia (section 3).

1. Risk Factors in Atherosclerosis

A risk factor for coronary heart disease (CHD) may be defined as an attribute which appears to occur more frequently among persons with CHD than among control subjects, although causality is not necessarily implied [1]. To this definition should be added the caveat that modification of the said attribute cannot be assumed to overcome or ease the risk of subsequently developing CHD. The recognition of risk factors on the one hand and the known benefits of intervention on the other will be considered separately.

Prospective population studies over the last 20 to 30 years have documented a long list of key risk factors associated with atherosclerosis. The contribution of certain major factors has been accepted unequivocally while others remain of uncertain significance. These risk factors have been grouped in table I.

Data from the National Co-operative Pooling Project (NCPP) in the USA suggest that 70 % of coronary heart disease cases (angina pectoris, myocardial infarction, sudden death) are attributable to three of the primary risk factors, cigarette smoking,

Table I. Key risk factors in atherosclerosis

---

1. *Primary (i.e. Independent) Risk Factors*
    Cigarette smoking
    Hypertension
    Hypercholesterolaemia
    Reduced HDL cholesterol concentration

2. *Secondary Risk Factors (? Primary in Some Cases)*
    Diabetes mellitus
    Hypertriglyceridaemia
    Obesity
    Physical inactivity
    Gout and hyperuricaemia
    Stress and personality type
    Family history of CHD

3. *Risk Factors of Uncertain Significance*
    Water hardness
    Carbohydrate and fibre intake

---

hypertension and hypercholesterolaemia, with each factor being of approximately equal importance [2]. The same risk factors are operative in cerebral atherosclerosis, although the relative weightings are different, hypertension appearing to be of paramount importance. In peripheral vascular disease, cigarette smoking, hypertriglyceridaemia and diabetes seem to be of importance.

Although the strength of the individual association may vary, the majority of atherosclerosis-related events can be attributed to one or more of the known risk factors. Other factors will be added in time. However, it is beyond the scope of the present work to consider the contributions of risk factors that are not closely related to lipids.

1.1 Hypercholesterolaemia

While a debate may rage as to the merits of *lowering* elevated plasma cholesterol levels, there is uniform agreement that hypercholesterolaemia is an important and primary risk factor in CHD [3-6]. The Framingham Study has demonstrated a linear increase in coronary risk with increments in total plasma cholesterol level from 180mg/100ml (4.7mmol/litre) upwards [7] (fig. 1).

Data of this type have suggested that any level of plasma cholesterol across the whole distribution is potentially atherogenic and theoretically desirable values might be those which are as low as possible. This could mean that more than half the population would need to follow aggressive dietary and drug therapy, entailing a catastrophic economic and social cost to the community.

Data from NCPP also support the importance of hypercholesterolaemia as a primary risk factor, but provide much less evidence of a linear relationship between vascular risk and cholesterol levels below 250mg/100ml (6.5mmol/litre) [8]. The risk doubles with cholesterol levels over 250mg/100ml and trebles with levels in excess of 300 (7.8mmol/litre). This suggests that individuals whose values exceed 250 might merit intervention. Whether an individual whose present cholesterol level is 235 (6.1mmol/litre) would benefit by having it lowered to below 200 (5.2mmol/litre) is not known.

These comments concerning absolute plasma cholesterol values refer only to mature adults in the particular study populations. Let us assume for the purposes of the present discussion that cholesterols are measured with similar methods and precision in Framingham, Sydney and Auckland, and further that the findings in a North American population can be transposed to Australia or New Zealand. It should be noted that the various assumptions are not entirely justified.

It is known that plasma cholesterol levels begin to rise from birth, show a slight depression in the mid-teens and then experience a further rise with adulthood [8,9]. Although a number of studies have evaluated lipid levels in children, as yet there are

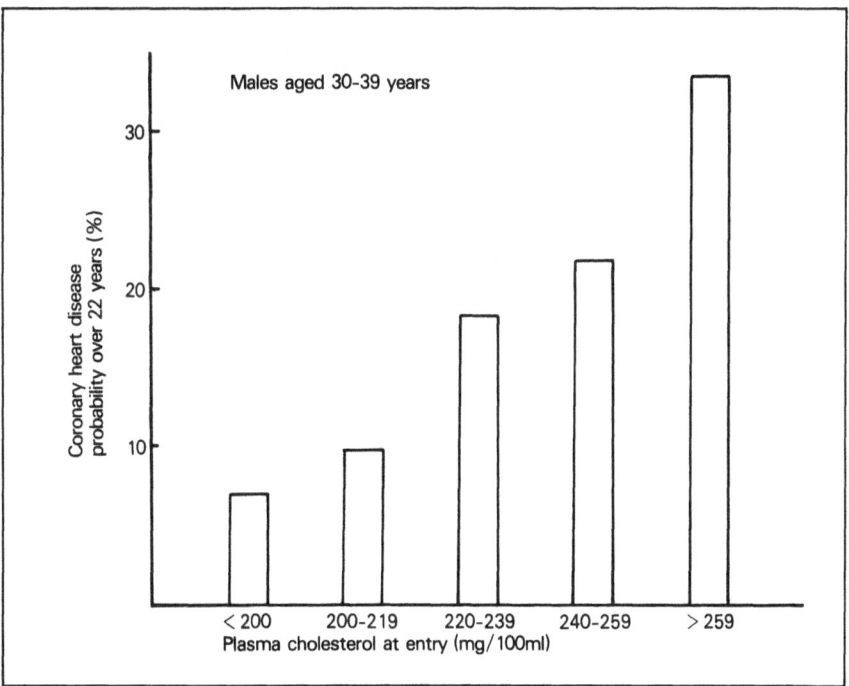

Fig. 1. Probability of developing coronary heart disease in relation to plasma cholesterol concentration at entry into the Framingham Study (modified from [7]).

no prospective data which allow one to determine 'safe' or desirable cholesterol values in this group.

Familial Hypercholesterolaemia

Aetiology of the hypercholesterolaemia may be of special significance in the association with vascular disease. For example, familial hypercholesterolaemia (FH) is a disorder which has been clearly linked with CHD.

FH is an autosomal dominant trait, is completely penetrant but with variable expression, and is the best understood of all the genetic hyperlipidaemias. It has an estimated frequency in the population of the USA and UK of about 0.2 % [10]. Defining all hypercholesterolaemia as those subjects above the 95th percentile, a very arbitrary and conservative approach, then only one in 25 of all hypercholesterolaemic subjects would have familial hypercholesterolaemia.

Slack has estimated that heterozygous males with FH, by the age of 50 years, have a 51.4 % chance of developing CHD and a 23.5 % expectation of coronary death. Females with FH have a 12.2 % chance of developing CHD by the age of 50 years [11]. The mean age of male myocardial infarct survivors with FH in Seattle, USA was 46 years, compared with 63 years among non-hyperlipidaemic infarct survivors. About 3 to 6 % of unselected middle-aged survivors of myocardial infarction in the USA and UK (and probably Australia) will have the genetic trait FH in the heterozygous form [12].

Homozygous subjects with FH are rarely found in the general population. This condition occurs with an apparent frequency of about one in one million [10]. Such patients experience extremely severe atherosclerosis and survival beyond 30 years of age has not been recorded. In these subjects there can be no doubt as to the causal relationship between FH and atherosclerosis.

Familial hypercholesterolaemia however is but one variety of hypercholesterolaemia. Here the risk factor is usually severe and of lifetime duration. Other members of the community may have similar plasma cholesterol levels (e.g. 300-350mg/100ml) not due to FH and may not necessarily have the very bad prognosis described above.

1.2 Dietary Cholesterol as a Risk Factor

A notable omission from the list of atherosclerosis risk factors in table I is dietary cholesterol. Misplaced enthusiasm in the mass media has led the layperson and some doctors to believe that hypercholesterolaemia has arisen solely through the ingestion of excessive amounts of cholesterol and that dietary cholesterol is the major cause of heart disease. In fact, patients with coronary heart disease within a given community have *not* been shown to differ significantly in their previous dietary habits from a comparable group without CHD [13]. Furthermore, there is little correlation between dietary cholesterol intake and plasma cholesterol concentration within homogeneous population groups (see page 7).

It would be incorrect to discount any role for diet in the causation of CHD. For instance, various populations have shown a reduced CHD death rate and less severe coronary atherosclerosis at autopsy during wartime and food shortages [14]. Certain populations with an increased prevalence of CHD have a higher mean plasma cholesterol level than populations with a low CHD rate, while CHD rates and plasma cholesterol levels are both directly correlated with saturated fat in the diet [6]. None of these examples can be regarded as final evidence of a causal relationship between diet and coronary heart disease, since the prevalence of other risk factors may be changing concurrently.

1.3 Multiple Risk Factors

Prospective data from several studies indicate that combinations of the primary risk factors lead to an additive risk [15] (fig. 2). The presence of multiple risk factors

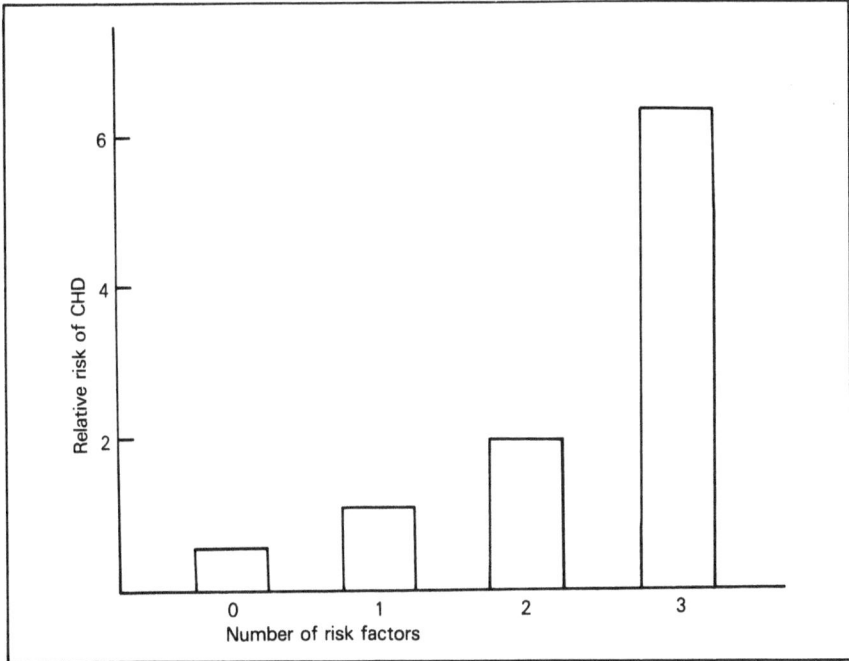

Fig. 2. Relative risk of developing coronary heart disease in relation to the number of risk factors present. The risk factors are plasma cholesterol > 250mg/100ml, systolic blood pressure > 159mm Hg and cigarette smoking > 20/day (modified from the Framingham Study data, [15]).

Table II. Incidence rate of CHD over 4 years by HDL cholesterol level in Framingham[1]

HDL cholesterol (mg/100ml)	Men (%)	Women (%)
< 25	17.7	—
25 — 34	10.0	16.4
35 — 44	10.5	5.5
45 — 54	5.1	4.9
55 — 64	6.0	4.0
65 — 74	2.5	1.4
75 +	—	2.0

1 Expressed as percent of population at risk (modified from [19]).

— combinations of high cholesterol levels, high blood pressure or cigarette smoking
— implies an unacceptably high level of risk and it is in this high risk group that treatment of hyperlipidaemia appears most strongly indicated [16].

Precise figures have been derived from the Framingham Study which have allowed the attending physician to predict the probability of a coronary event within a defined period of time in an individual patient [17]. While this approach correctly emphasises the additive effects of multiple risk factors, caution should be exercised in the general use of such tables. Their use implies a number of assumptions which are quantitatively unjustified, e.g. precise extrapolation of Framingham risk to other geographic centres, assumption of similar methodology and precision for clinical and biochemical measurements.

1.4 High Density Lipoprotein, a Negative or Protective Factor

Although lipoprotein quantitation and typing has been popular for almost 15 years, it was repeatedly asserted that a lipoprotein profile conferred little additional advantage over cholesterol estimation alone. This position has completely changed since 1975 when Miller and Miller refocused attention on *reduced* HDL cholesterol level as a possible risk factor [18]. This had first been suggested in 1951.

Women have much less premature CHD than males even in the presence of FH with comparable degrees of hypercholesterolaemia. It is known that premenopausal women have higher HDL levels than males. It is now suggested that variations in HDL cholesterol level may account for much of the difference in CHD incidence rates, both between the sexes and within the sexes. Prospective studies in Framingham over 4 years showed HDL cholesterol to be a negative or protective risk factor for future CHD, independently of all other factors for all age groups (table II). The incidence of CHD was noted to fall with increasing HDL levels and for comparable HDL levels the incidence rates for both the sexes were quite similar [19].

A number of studies over a comparatively short period of time have confirmed this negative relationship of HDL with coronary heart disease [20-23]. A similar relationship has also been shown to exist in patients with cerebral atherosclerosis [24]. The syndrome of familial hyperalphalipoproteinaemia (increased HDL levels) is associated with marked longevity and lends further weight to the protective role of HDL in atherosclerosis [25]. A potential biochemical basis for this protective role is presented on page 17.

In reference to hypercholesterolaemia as a risk factor, no mention was made of LDL or beta lipoprotein as the risk factor. Since the bulk of plasma cholesterol is transported in LDL, either LDL cholesterol or total plasma cholesterol may be taken as a valid expression of risk. The Framingham Study has derived a relationship between CHD risk and the ratio of plasma cholesterol to HDL cholesterol (table III). This ratio expresses mathematically the apparent biological interaction between the two lipoprotein classes LDL and HDL, an increasing ratio indicating greater CHD risk [26].

Further support for the use of an expression relating LDL to HDL comes from studies in vegetarians. Seventh Day Adventist vegetarians are known to have a low incidence of premature CHD [27] and actually have relatively low levels of HDL compared with non-vegetarians (table IV). However, their reduced HDL level is also accompanied by a favourably low LDL and total cholesterol level as well as by a low prevalence of other major risk factors [8].

The focus of attention on HDL and other lipoprotein classes is clearly the most significant advance in cardiovascular epidemiology in the last 10 years. The state of the art is changing rapidly and it is not considered prudent to make dogmatic statements as to the precise relationship of HDL and other lipoproteins to vascular disease.

Table III. Relationship of CHD to the ratio of total plasma cholesterol: HDL cholesterol [26]

CHD risk	Ratio in men	Ratio in women
Half average	3.43	3.29
Average	4.97	4.44
Twice average	9.55	7.05
Three times average	23.39	11.04

1.5 Hypertriglyceridaemia

It was suggested in table I that hypertriglyceridaemia is a secondary risk factor, although a primary role could not be excluded. Studies in Scandinavia have demonstrated a primary relationship between increased triglyceride levels and CHD risk, independently of other risk factors such as cholesterol.

The Stockholm Prospective Study failed to demonstrate a continuous gradient between triglyceride concentration and CHD risk [4], although the 15-year follow-up data clearly show increased risk at the highest level of triglyceride concentration. Recent results from Finland in males 50 to 53 years old suggest a similar finding, with increased cardiovascular mortality at triglyceride concentrations in excess of 1.7mmol/litre, independently of the cholesterol concentrations (fig. 3) [28]. The lack

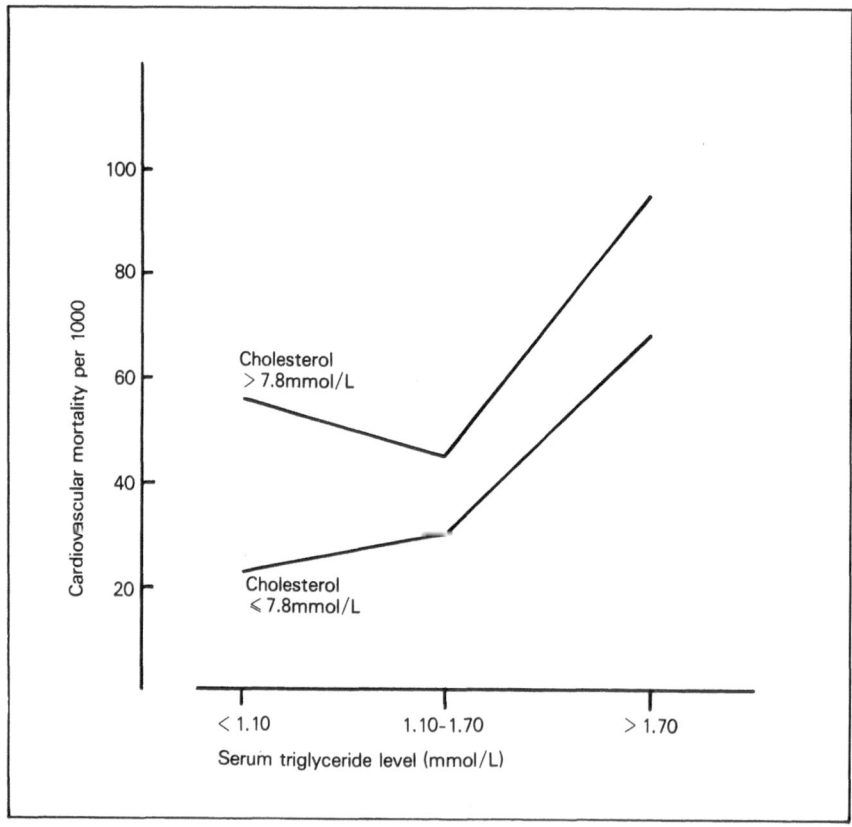

Fig. 3. Cardiovascular mortality in relation to serum triglyceride levels in Finnish males. Data corrected for cholesterol concentration (from [28] with the kind permission of the authors and editors).

Table IV. A comparison of HDL and total cholesterol values in Seventh Day Adventist vegetarians and non-vegetarian controls[1]

Subjects	Plasma cholesterol (mg/100ml)	HDL cholesterol (mg/100ml)	Total cholesterol: HDL cholesterol
Vegetarians (n = 45)	164 ± 21[2]	40 ± 7[2]	4.10
Controls (n = 48)	204 ± 31	46 ± 7	4.43

1 Age-matched control subjects drawn from the Sydney Coronary Heart Disease Prevention Programme. Male subjects only considered. Mean ± S.D.
2 Significantly different from controls by t-test, $p < 0.01$.

of a continuous gradient of risk with increasing triglyceride levels contrasts with the example of cholesterol and other primary risk factors and is difficult to explain.

Other studies have shown an increase in CHD risk with increasing triglyceride levels, yet this risk could largely be explained by association with other factors such as hypercholesterolaemia, reduced HDL, obesity and diabetes. Hypertriglyceridaemia is clearly a significant risk factor in vascular disease, whether primary or secondary, and routine measurement is justified. It is suggested that a plasma triglyceride concentration in excess of 180mg/100ml (2.0mmol/litre) would justify intervention.

1.6 Other Risk Factors Possibly Related to Lipids

Other risk factors listed in table I may influence atherosclerosis directly, or indirectly through association at least in part, with abnormalities in lipid and lipoprotein metabolism.

Obesity and physical inactivity are important and probably inter-related risk factors. Both have been linked with reduced HDL cholesterol levels [29] while obese subjects often have evidence of hyperlipidaemia, high blood pressure and occasionally diabetes mellitus. Life insurance data show a steady increase in excess mortality as relative weight increases and most of this excess mortality is from cardiovascular disease. Any argument as to whether obesity is a primary or secondary risk factor is a semantic one because of the pivotal role attributed to overweight in the management of hyperlipidaemia.

Diabetes mellitus is associated at times with the same type of macroscopic atherosclerosis as is noted in the presence of other major risk factors. The occurrence of this complication is probably related to the duration of the diabetes and supposedly is a manifestation of poor control. Diabetic subjects may show marked hypertriglyceridaemia and reduced HDL cholesterol [30]. This finding is not universal and there are probably better markers of diabetic control.

Most epidemiological studies have highlighted the association of gout, hyperuricaemia and CHD. Gout and hyperuricaemia are also associated with hypertriglyceridaemia and obesity. Despite the strength of these associations, no strong argument has been advanced in favour of lowering urate levels to prevent CHD.

The relationship of stress and CHD is a vexed question. Personality type A, characterised by enhanced aggressiveness, ambition, competitive drive and a chronic sense of time urgency, is associated with about twice as much CHD as type B, independently of any change in other risk factors [31]. Type A subjects show a trend towards slightly higher lipid values and this relationship is currently under investigation.

Primitive populations show very little CHD, while they maintain a simple diet rich in vegetable fibre, a class of complex non-digestible polysaccharide. Western man ingests much less dietary fibre by comparison and the hypothesis has been advanced that a diet low in fibre constitutes a CHD risk factor [32]. This effect is supposedly mediated through cholesterol metabolism, perhaps through interference with the enterohepatic circulation of bile salts. Laboratory investigation and clinical trials have not substantiated early claims in this regard and the fibre story must remain hypothetical for the present.

2. Abdominal Pain, Pancreatitis and Hyperlipidaemia

Severe upper abdominal pain, with or without documentable acute pancreatitis, is an *occasional* accompaniment of severe hypertriglyceridaemia. In general this will not arise unless the triglyceride concentration exceeds approximately 20mmol/litre. This is found in the presence of the extremely rare type I hyperlipoproteinaemia or the relatively more common type V hyperlipoproteinaemia [33] (chapter IV, 2.1).

The serum from a patient with type V hyperlipoproteinaemia has a characteristic creamy appearance due to the presence of large lipoprotein particles, chylomicrons and VLDL. If this is observed in the presence of an acute abdomen, then a conservative approach is indicated in the first instance and unless there are additional indications for surgery, exploratory laparotomy should be postponed. The cause of the acute abdominal pain with hypertriglyceridaemia is uncertain. Some of the patients have diagnosable acute pancreatitis, by virtue of increased urinary amylase excretion. Determination of serum amylase tends to be unreliable in the presence of extreme serum turbidity and may at times be non-diagnostic, even with clear serum.

One point is very certain in these patients — attacks of abdominal pain are precipitated by ingestion of fat and do not occur if the dietary intake of fat is severely restricted. Hypertriglyceridaemia and abdominal pain are absolute indications for antihyperlipidaemia therapy.

3. Cutaneous Manifestations of Hyperlipidaemia

Cutaneous signs of hyperlipidaemia are sometimes present and occasionally require local treatment. More often these signs serve as markers of underlying metabolic disorders, without requiring local treatment.

External signs of hyperlipidaemia include the premature corneal arcus (under 55 years), xanthelasmata around the eyelids, tendon xanthomata (hands, elbows, ankles and feet), tuberous xanthomata (pressure areas near knees, buttocks, ankles and elbows), palmar xanthomata and eruptive xanthomata (also pressure areas). Arcus and xanthelasmata may occasionally be found in young subjects without apparent hyperlipidaemia. When significant, they are usually evidence of hypercholesterolaemia. Tendon xanthomata are the hallmark of familial hypercholesterolaemia, while eruptive xanthomata usually signify massive hypertriglyceridaemia. Familial hypercholesterolaemic patients may occasionally have xanthomatous deposits in the small bones of the fingers and toes, with an x-ray appearance indistinguishable from gout.

With the possible exception of facial lesions, xanthomata do not usually create any local problems. With prolonged medical therapy it is usual for xanthomata, including facial lesions, to regress or at least stabilise in size. It has been fashionable to excise or apply local treatment to xanthelasmata. This practice is to be deprecated, as surgically treated lesions will rapidly return unless metabolic therapy is also offered.

Synopsis

Atherosclerosis-related events are associated with four primary or independent risk factors — cigarette smoking, high blood pressure, increased plasma cholesterol concentration and reduced HDL cholesterol concentration. These risk factors are particularly significant when present in combination. The dietary cholesterol intake by itself does not appear to be a risk factor. Hypertriglyceridaemia is also a vascular risk factor but it remains unclear whether this is independent of other factors. Other risk factors may also operate in part through associated changes in lipid metabolism.

Extreme hypertriglyceridaemia is associated with abdominal pain and pancreatitis. Such patients require conservative therapy in the first instance, as attacks of pain are precipitated by the ingestion of fat and are prevented by restricting fat intake.

Patients with hyperlipidaemia may occasionally have cutaneous manifestations including corneal arcus and xanthomata. These are signs of an underlying metabolic disorder and do not usually require local treatment. Cosmetic problems, if any, usually respond to medical therapy.

References

1. Epstein, F.H.: The epidemiology of coronary heart disease. A review. Journal of Chronic Diseases 18: 735-774 (1965)
2. Miettinen, O.S.: Risk indicators for coronary heart disease. Hartford Hospital Bulletin 4: 1964 (1973). Quoted by Whyte, H.M.: Australian and New Zealand Journal of Medicine 6: 387-393 (1976).
3. Kannel, W.B.; Castelli, W.P.; Gordon, T. and McNamara, P.H.: Serum cholesterol, lipoproteins and risk of coronary heart disease. The Framingham Study. Annals of Internal Medicine 74: 1-12 (1971).
4. Carlson, L.A. and Bottiger, L.E.: Ischaemic heart disease in relation to fasting values of plasma triglycerides and cholesterol. Lancet 1: 865-868 (1972).
5. Welborn, T.A.; Cumston, G.N.; Cullen, K.J.; Curnow, D.H.; McCall, M.G. and Stenhouse, N.S.: The prevalence of coronary heart disease and associated factors in an Australian rural community. American Journal of Epidemiology 89: 521-536 (1969).
6. Keys, A.: Coronary heart disease in seven countries. Circulation 41 (Suppl. 1) (1970).
7. Dawber, T.R.: Risk factors for atherosclerotic disease; In Current Medical Topics p.5-36 (The Upjohn Company, Michigan 1975).
8. Stamler, J.: Lifestyle, major risk factors, proof and public policy. Circulation 58: 3-19 (1978).
9. Morrison, J.A.; deGroot, I.; Edwards, B.K.; Kelly, K.A.; Rauh, J.L.; Mellies, M. and Glueck, C.J.: Plasma cholesterol and triglyceride levels in 6775 school children, ages 6-17. Metabolism 26: 1199-1211 (1977).
10. Motulsky, A.G.: Current concepts in genetics. The genetic hyperlipidemias. New England Journal of Medicine 294: 823-827 (1976).
11. Slack, J.: Risks of ischaemic heart disease in familial hyperlipoproteinaemic states. Lancet 2: 1380-1382 (1969).
12. Goldstein, J.L.; Hazzard, W.R.; Schrott, H.G.; Biermann, E.L.; and Motulsky, A.G.: Hyperlipidemia in coronary heart disease. I. Lipid levels in 500 survivors of myocardial infarction. II. Genetic analysis of lipid levels in 176 families and delineation of a new inherited disorder. III. Evaluation of lipoprotein phenotypes of 156 genetically defined survivors of myocardial infarction. Journal of Clinical Investigation 52: 1533-1577 (1973).
13. Coronary heart disease. A progress report, 1976. National Heart Foundation of New Zealand (1976).
14. Malmros, H.: The relation of nutrition to health. A statistical study of the effect of the wartime on arteriosclerosis, cardiosclerosis, tuberculosis and diabetes. Acta Med. Scand. (Suppl.) 246 (1950).
15. Gordon, T.; Sorlie, P. and Kannel, W.B. in The Framingham Study: An epidemiological investigation of cardiovascular disease. Section 27. (US Department of Health, Education and Welfare, National Institutes of Health, Maryland 1971).
16. Whyte, H.M.: Potential effect on coronary heart disease morbidity of lowering the blood cholesterol. Lancet 1: 906-910 (1975).
17. Coronary Risk Handbook: Estimating risk of coronary heart disease in daily practice. (American Heart Association, New York 1973).
18. Miller, G.J. and Miller, N.E.: Plasma high density lipoprotein concentration and development of ischaemic heart disease. Lancet 1: 16-19 (1975).
19. Gordon, T.; Castelli, W.P.; Hjortland, M.C.; Kannel, W.B. and Dawber, T.R.: High density lipoproteins as a protective factor against coronary heart disease. The Framingham Study. American Journal of Medicine 62: 707-714 (1977).
20. Miller, N.E.; Forde, O.H.; Thelle, D.S. and Mjos, O.D.: The Tromso Heart Study. High density lipoprotein and coronary heart disease: A prospective case-controlled study. Lancet 1: 965-968 (1977).

21. Castelli, W.P.; Doyle, J.T.; Gordon, T.; Hames, C.; Hjortland, M.C.; Hulley, S.B.; Kagan, A. and
     Zukel, W.J.: HDL cholesterol and other lipids in coronary heart disease. The Co-operative Lipopro-
     tein Phenotyping Study. Circulation 55: 767-772 (1977).
22. Miller, G.J.; Miller, N.E. and Ashcroft, M.T.: Inverse relationship in Jamaica between plasma high
     density lipoprotein cholesterol concentration and coronary disease risk as predicted by multiple risk
     factor status. Clinical Science and Molecular Medicine 51: 475-482 (1976).
23. Sammel, N.; Simons, L.A.; Hickie, J.B. and Gibson J.C.: Coronary artery disease in young
     Australian women. Medical Journal of Australia 2: 495-497 (1978).
24. Rossner, S.; Mettinger, K.L.; Kjellin, K.G.; Mettinger, K.L., Siden, A. and Soderstrom, C.E.: Nor-
     mal serum cholesterol but low HDL cholesterol concentration in young patients with ischaemic
     cerebro-vascular disease. Lancet 1: 577-579 (1978).
25. Glueck, C.J.; Fallat, R.W.; Millet, F.; Gartside, P.; Elston, R.C. and Go, R.C.: Familial hyperalpha-
     lipoproteinemia. Metabolism 24: 1253-1266 (1975).
26. Castelli, W.P.: HDL in assessing risk of coronary heart disease. Guidelines to Metabolic Therapy 6:
     No. 3 (The Upjohn Company, Michigan 1977).
27. Phillips, R.L.; Lemon, F.R.; Beeson, W.L. and Kuzma, J.W.: Coronary heart disease mortality
     among Seventh-Day Adventists with differing dietary habits: A preliminary report. American Jour-
     nal of Clinical Nutrition 31: 191-198 (1978).
28. Pelkonen, R.; Nikkila, E.A.; Koskinen, S.; Penttinen, K. and Savna, S.: Association of serum lipids
     and obesity with cardiovascular mortality. British Medical Journal 2: 1185-1187 (1977).
29. Wood, P.D.; Haskell, W.; Klein, H.; Lewis, S.; Stern, M. and Farquhar, J.W.: The distribution of
     plasma lipoproteins in middle aged runners. Metabolism 25: 1249-1257 (1976).
30. Lopes-Virella, M.F.L.; Stone, P.G. and Colwell, J.A.: Serum high density lipoprotein in diabetic
     patients. Diabetologia 13: 285-291 (1977).
31. Rosenman, R.H.; Brand, R.J.; Jenkins, C.D.; Friedman, M.; Straus, R. and Wurm, M.: Coronary
     heart disease in the Western Collaborative Group Study. Journal of the American Medical Associa-
     tion 233: 872-877 (1975).
32. Trowell, H.: Ischemic heart disease and dietary fiber. American Journal of Clinical Nutrition 25:
     926-932 (1972).
33. Simons, L.A.; Williams; P.F. and Turtle, J.R.: Type V hyperlipoproteinaemia re-visited: Findings
     in a Sydney population. Australian and New Zealand Journal of Medicine 5: 210-219 (1975).

Chapter III

Is Risk Factor Intervention Worthwhile?

Since the atherosclerotic process continues during the entire lifetime of the individual, any intervention begun late in life might be expected to achieve only limited benefit. The degree of benefit achieved would be expected to be related to the relative effectiveness of the lowering in plasma cholesterol, blood pressure and so on, but would also be related to the time in life when the requisite changes were introduced. These considerations make it imperative to begin intervention as early as possible and to achieve as much modification as possible, *but without causing harm.*

1. Atherosclerosis in Different Anatomical Sites

In the discussion of atherosclerosis risk factors in chapter II, little emphasis was placed on the actual anatomical sites of the lesions. Most attention was focused on CHD and it was assumed that a similar pattern of risk factors operated in cases of cerebral arteriosclerosis, carotid arterial disease and peripheral vascular disease involving the abdominal aorta and vessels of the lower limbs. In fact, the risk factor profile for non-CHD atherosclerosis is much the same, differing only in the relative weightings of individual factors.

Hypercholesterolaemia and reduced HDL cholesterol remain of some importance in all anatomical sites of atherosclerosis. However, cigarette smoking will have been observed by all clinicians to have had a particularly dramatic effect on peripheral ischaemic symptoms, as well as on peripheral disease progression. Hypertensive intracranial haemorrhage might be regarded, in part, as a complication of intra-cerebral atherosclerosis. High blood pressure is certainly regarded as a key risk factor in this setting, whether or not the atherosclerotic process is influenced. Hypertriglyceridaemia is often stated to be a most important risk factor in peripheral vascular disease.

Although they are no doubt associated, this relationship requires confirmation by prospective study, most of the published studies having been performed in a retro-spective manner in selected patients.

Most of the worldwide effort in cardiovascular epidemiology and risk factor modification has been focused on CHD, mainly because the case numbers far exceed all other clinical manifestations of atherosclerosis. As a result, a large body of knowledge is available in relation to CHD and much less is known in relation to the other areas. The remaining discussion in this chapter will reflect this balance of knowledge.

2. Regression of Atherosclerosis

In the presence of advanced atherosclerosis, end-organ damage may already be apparent, e.g. myocardial or cerebral infarction. Under these circumstances the ulti-mate prognosis would be unlikely to show improvement through any potential regression in the atherosclerotic lesions.

The very nature of advanced and complicated atheroma, showing a localised pic-ture of ulceration, thrombosis, tissue necrosis, calcification and cholesterol crystalli-sation, suggests that this stage of the disease is irreversible. In regard to less advanced atheroma, there is clear evidence in animals and meagre evidence in man that lesions may be reversible. Monkeys who have hypercholesterolaemia induced by relatively short term feeding of human types of diet, rich in cholesterol and saturated fats (uncharacteristic for the animal), develop lesions of a human type, which may com-pletely regress with return of the animal to its habitual diet and habitual cholesterol level [1]. Evidence for regression of lesions in man is less convincing, although early pre-symptomatic femoral atherosclerosis has been shown to regress following suc-cessful management of hyperlipidaemia and hypertension [2].

In the absence of hard evidence of regression of atherosclerosis, the aims of therapy in clinical practice are restricted to the prevention of lesions and to the arrest of further progress. In addition, the ultimate clinical outcome may not be closely linked to progression of atheromatous lesions. Instead it may be linked to a specific complication such as thrombosis. In this context, a number of therapeutic agents which may influence blood coagulation are under intensive investigation (e.g. aspirin, dipyridamole and sulphinpyrazone), in the areas of CHD, peripheral vascular disease and cerebrovascular disease.

3. Primary *Versus* Secondary Prevention

Primary prevention of atherosclerosis refers to risk factor intervention in sub-jects showing no overt evidence of vascular disease, as judged by non-invasive methods. Routine coronary arteriography in patients with risk factors would un-

Table I. Probability of developing CHD in 20 years for young men. Potential benefits from lowering plasma cholesterol (modified from [7])

Plasma cholesterol	Probability (%)	
	Low risk[1]	High risk[2]
310mg/100ml	14	57
210mg/100ml	5	28
Potential benefit		
310 → 210mg/100ml	9	29

1 Low risk = non-smoker, systolic blood pressure 120mmHg, no ECG abnormality.
2 High risk = cigarette smoker, systolic blood pressure 165mmHg, left ventricular hypertrophy (ECG).

doubtedly reveal many more subjects with significant coronary artery disease who do not have clinical manifestations. Secondary prevention refers to management of patients who already have clinical manifestations of vascular disease.

Secondary prevention has been practised in trials and in clinical medicine for many years because such patients are numerous and have strong motivation. Secondary prevention intervention on behalf of lipids has been generally unrewarding (with certain exceptions to be discussed later in this chapter).

Intervention for cigarette smoking and hypertension in the contexts of both primary and secondary prevention has been shown to be of undisputed clinical benefit. Smokers under 65 years of age who give up smoking rapidly lose their increased vascular risk [3], whilst survival after myocardial infarction is significantly improved in the ex-smokers compared with patients who continue to smoke [4]. Treated hypertensives have a significantly reduced incidence of cerebral haemorrhage and atherothrombotic brain infarction [5], while also having a lower incidence of congestive cardiac failure. Although early studies suggested that reduction in blood pressure did not reduce the subsequent rate of myocardial infarction, one recent study has shown that such therapy might indeed reduce the infarction rate [6].

4. Who to Treat

The question of who to treat for hyperlipidaemia (or any other major risk factor) is best answered as ... 'those subjects at greatest cardiovascular risk'. These are patients with multiple risk factors.

Table II. Major coronary events, rates per 1,000 subjects per annum, in the WHO clofibrate trial [8]

Quartile of Risk Score	Clofibrate	Placebo	Difference
1 (lowest risk)	1.11	2.51	1.40
2	4.70	5.18	0.48
3	6.58	9.47	2.89
4 (highest risk)	12.56	16.25	3.72

Whyte [7] has examined this question in a perceptive analysis of the Framingham data, making the important assumption that a sizable reduction in serum cholesterol (e.g. 310 to 210mg/100ml) confers upon the subject a reduced but still finite level of risk (table I). 29% of males aged 35 years in the high risk category (multiple risk factors) might benefit by cholesterol reduction from 310 to 210, whereas only 9% of males in the low risk category (single risk factor) would similarly derive benefit. 28% of high risk males would still suffer a coronary event despite cholesterol lowering. This raises a vital issue: it is unreasonable to expect total prevention of CHD. One may reasonably expect reduction of the incidence rate to a lower but still finite level.

A recently completed primary prevention trial with clofibrate, which will be discussed later, illustrates that intervention for cholesterol in the presence of multiple risk factors is more than a hypothetical concept [8]. Although this study failed to reduce the death rate from CHD, an overall 25% reduction in the non-fatal myocardial infarction rate was noted. Maximum benefit was clearly obtained in subjects in the highest quartiles of risk, i.e. those with multiple risk factors (table II).

·5. Dietary Intervention For Cholesterol

It is accepted that reduction in the intake of cholesterol and saturated fats and an increased intake of polyunsaturated fats (primarily linoleic acid) are capable of significantly reducing the plasma cholesterol level. This dietary approach has formed the basis of numerous intervention trials.

Between 1965 and 1977 at least nine dietary intervention studies have been reported, four being primary prevention in type. The implications of most of these studies have been reviewed by the National Heart Foundation of Australia and a working party of the Australian Academy of Science [9,10]. In essence, dietary intervention in the presence of existing CHD had no consistent effect on mortality, although it may have reduced morbidity. Primary prevention trials with diet seemed to reduce CHD mortality rates in younger subjects, if not total mortality. Four key illustrative studies will be discussed in detail, the first three concerning primary or mixed primary-secondary prevention, and the fourth secondary prevention.

The Finnish Mental Hospital Study in Helsinki administered this type of diet for 6 years in turn, in each of 2 hospitals, comparing the results with a standard diet [11]. In males 35 to 65 years of age, the fat-modified diet was associated with significantly reduced mortality from CHD, with a similar although not significant trend in total mortality. The Los Angeles Veterans Trial was a double-blind trial in males aged 54 to 89 years, undertaken over 7 years, using a fat-modified diet [12]. A significant reduction in cardiovascular mortality was observed only in subjects under 65 years of age, with a trend towards lower total mortality which was not significant.

Another intervention involving encouragement of dietary changes in large free-living populations was performed in Belgium [13]. Between 1960 and 1971 the diet in north Belgium was lower in cholesterol and saturated fats and higher in polyunsaturates compared with the south. Mean serum cholesterol levels by 1968-1969 were 10 to 12mg/100ml lower in the north compared with the south and this was associated with a 25% lower total and cardiovascular mortality in males aged 25 to 64 years. It is also important to note that the fat-modified diet consumed in the north was not associated with an increased incidence of other serious diseases such as cancer.

The Sydney Diet Heart Study [14] offered a fat-modified, polyunsaturated enriched diet to male myocardial infarct survivors, aged 30 to 59 years, over a 2 to 7-year follow-up period. Control subjects followed a diet with partial fat modification. Despite a favourable influence on plasma lipid levels, there was no significant difference in survival between the two groups. This result essentially confirmed earlier findings in a UK study [15].

These various dietary intervention studies have their shortcomings. The Finnish Study was performed in mentally ill patients in hospital, the duration of hospital residence was variable, subjects were not well randomised and the design was not double blind. The Los Angeles trial used relatively elderly subjects, dietary adherence was sometimes poor and hence the total composition of the diet was unknown. The Belgian Study did not report the actual changes in mortality in the north over the 10-year period, but rather contrasted absolute death rates with those in the south, assuming that populations in the north and south were fully comparable. In the Sydney Diet Heart Study both patient groups underwent some dietary modification.

Despite these shortcomings, a general conclusion still emerges — male subjects under 65 years and free of CHD, consuming a cholesterol-lowering diet, seem to have a significantly lower CHD mortality and tend towards a lower total mortality. No firmer conclusion can be drawn from these studies, although one might speculate as to the outcome of similar studies performed in patients with hypercholesterolaemia and other risk factors.

After consideration of all the epidemiological and dietary intervention data various national committees have expressed the view that there is a case for a prudent fat-modified diet in some, if not all, members of the population [16-18]. There are individual scientists who hold dissenting views.

6. Drug Therapy for Hyperlipidaemia

A number of important trials to evaluate the role of lipid-lowering drugs in CHD prevention have been completed or are still in progress. Most attention has been focused on cholesterol lowering, while little information is available about the benefits of triglyceride reduction.

A 5-year double-blind trial of clofibrate in males with pre-existing CHD was reported from Edinburgh and Newcastle-upon-Tyne in 1971 [19,20]. Patients with pre-existing angina treated with clofibrate (but not those with previous infarction alone) showed a significant reduction in the number of fatal and non-fatal infarcts, the maximal effect being in the group 'sudden death'. This protection with clofibrate seemed to be unrelated to the observed effects on plasma lipids and remains unexplained.

Krasno and Kidera in 1972 reported an essentially primary prevention trial in males taking clofibrate [21]. With a single-blind technique over 39 months, the non-fatal myocardial infarction rate was significantly lower in the subjects on active therapy, 1.89 per 1,000 per year *versus* 6.6, although there was no significant difference in mortality rates between the active and placebo groups.

The Coronary Drug Project was a double-blind trial in male survivors of myocardial infarction utilising one of four therapeutic agents: oestrogens, dextrothyroxine, nicotinic acid (niacin) and clofibrate. Excessive mortality in the active treatment group necessitated premature termination of patients on oestrogens or thyroxine, but the 6-year experience with clofibrate and nicotinic acid was reported in 1975 [22]. Neither drug had any significant influence on total mortality rates comparing active therapy with placebo, although a trend towards fewer non-fatal re-infarctions was observed in the nicotinic acid treated group.

This carefully performed investigation has been criticised on the grounds that the serum cholesterol decrement produced by therapy (10 % with nicotinic acid and 6 % with clofibrate) was insufficient to be helpful in patients with established atherosclerosis. Carlson et al. [23] have reported preliminary results from an open trial in similar patients who were treated more aggressively with a combination of nicotinic acid and clofibrate, where a 15 to 20 % reduction in cholesterol and a 30 % reduction in triglycerides was observed. Over 3 to 4 years no significant difference in total mortality has emerged between drug and control groups, but the rate of non-fatal re-infarction was reduced by 50 % in the nicotinic acid and clofibrate treated group (fig. 1).

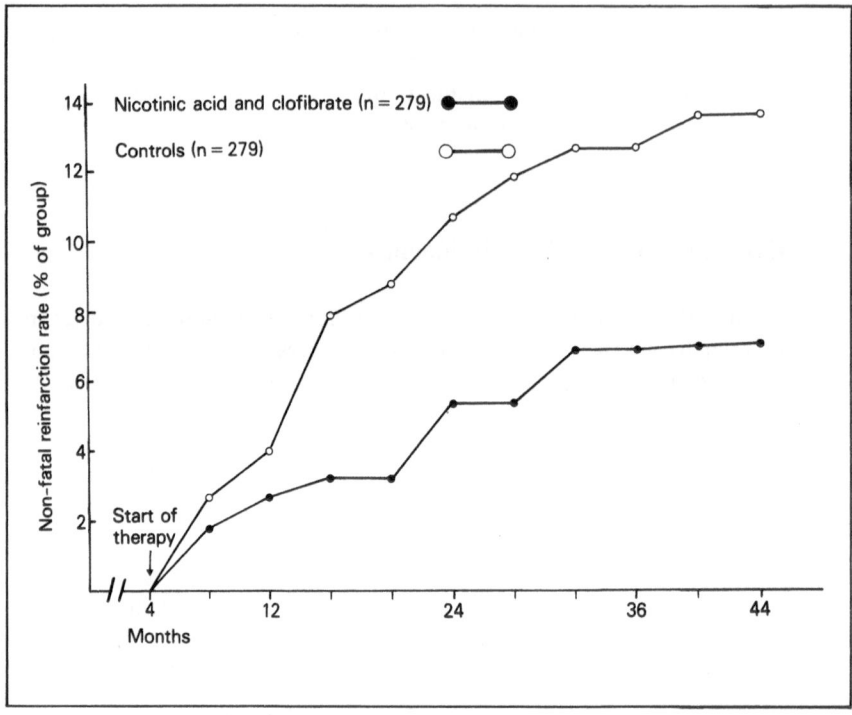

Fig. 1. Cumulative incidence of non-fatal re-infarction in Stockholm males treated with nicotinic acid and clofibrate compared with untreated controls (modified from [23] with kind permission of the authors and editor).

The last trial to be considered in this group is a single-blind study over 3 years with the new anion-exchange resin, colestipol [24]. For an average 12% fall in plasma cholesterol, male subjects with pre-existing CHD had significantly lower total and CHD mortality rates when treated with colestipol, compared with placebo. This effect was largely confined to patients under the age of 50 years, those with cholesterol values more than 299mg/100ml and triglycerides more than 149mg/100ml. No significant difference in mortality rate between colestipol and placebo treated groups was noted in women or in male patients without pre-existing CHD. However, the spontaneous number of CHD events in this last category would have been too few to discern any difference, if present.

As with the major dietary intervention trials, criticisms exist with respect to the drug intervention studies. For example, the Edinburgh-Newcastle studies contained some discordant results which have been largely overlooked by the pooling of findings from the separate trials; Krasno and Kidera employed a non-random allocation of patients to treatment groups; the Coronary Drug Project failed to produce 'substantial' serum lipid lowering; Carlson et al. did not appear to use a placebo in the control group; the colestipol study lacked uniform criteria for CHD in the different study centres and the rate of withdrawal from both active and placebo groups was very high at about 38 % overall. Finally, the majority of patients used in these studies had pre-existing CHD, which might argue against a favourable outcome.

Certain qualified conclusions still emerge from these studies. In secondary prevention studies, it seems that the use of lipid-lowering drugs may be associated with a lower non-fatal re-infarction rate, provided a substantial decrement in serum lipids results. Effects of this therapy on CHD mortality are more difficult to demonstrate.

6.1 Primary Prevention with Lipid-lowering Drugs

The major question . . . 'is risk factor intervention for lipids worthwhile?' may never be unequivocally answered, because each carefully planned investigation seems to produce new criticism and new questions. Some answers should be forthcoming from primary prevention trials still in progress.

Two major intervention programmes for primary hypercholesterolaemia are now underway in the USA. The Cholestyramine Lipid Research Clinic Trial is an example of single risk factor intervention, while the Multiple Risk Factor Intervention Trial also offers management of hypertension, cigarette smoking and physical inactivity [25]. Other multiple risk factor intervention programmes are underway in Europe [26] and Scandinavia [27]. These studies are still several years from completion.

The WHO European Primary Prevention Trial with clofibrate has recently presented its findings [8]. Males aged 30 to 59 years at entry and free of CHD, were drawn from the top one-third of population cholesterol values. Approximately 5,000 subjects were enrolled in a group to receive clofibrate and a similar number of matched subjects received a placebo in a double-blind fashion. Another group of approximately 5,000, drawn from the lower one-third of population cholesterol values, served as a further 'low cholesterol' control. About 68 % of subjects completed at least 5 years of follow-up.

Clofibrate therapy was associated with a significant 25 % reduction in the rate of non-fatal myocardial infarction, while the cardiovascular mortality rate remained disappointingly unaltered (fig. 2). Reduction in the infarction rate was most prominent in subjects with highest cholesterol values at entry, those with the largest serum cholesterol decrement and in those with multiple risk factors (see table II).

This trial produced some disquieting features. The cholecystectomy rate for gallstones was significantly increased in the treated group, although still at a very low level. This effect has been described in previous clofibrate trials [22] and in trials using polyunsaturated fats [28]. Furthermore, there was an excess number of deaths in the active treatment group from diseases of the gallbladder, liver and intestine, including malignant neoplasms of these sites. The numbers concerned here were very small and

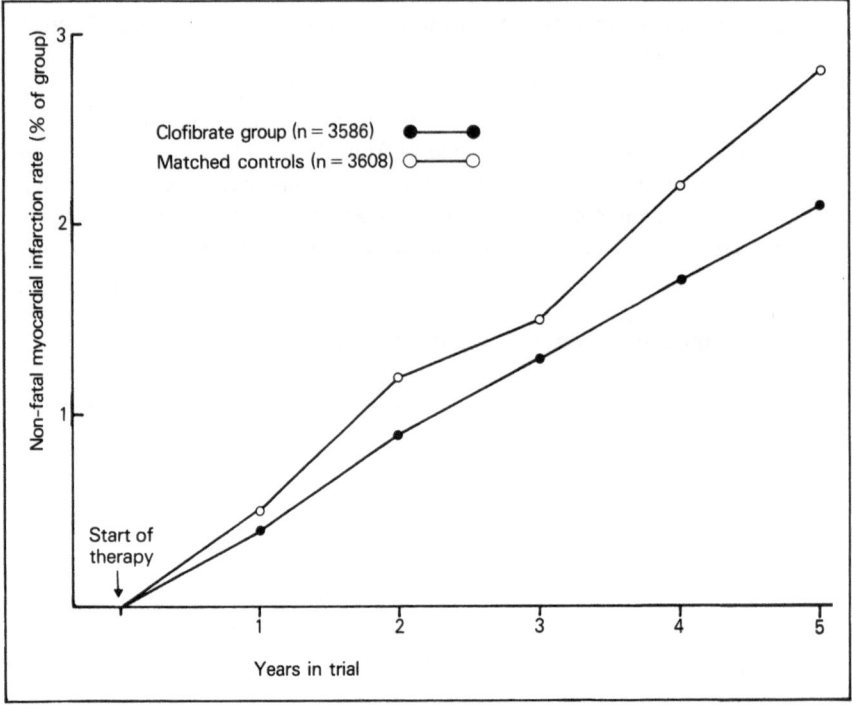

Fig. 2. Cumulative non-fatal myocardial infarction rate in males treated with clofibrate in the WHO trial (modified from [8] with kind permission of the authors and editor).

this may have been a chance finding. This important observation was not made in earlier equally well performed clofibrate trials [19,20,22] and therefore should not occasion immediate alarm. However, even if this is a remote possiblility, then clofibrate should be reserved for cases of definite hyperlipidaemia not responding to dietary or other measures.

These results have perhaps posed as many questions for the future as have already been answered. The improvement in non-fatal infarction rate is a similar finding to that observed in the secondary prevention studies already discussed. At face value, lipid lowering with clofibrate does not reduce the CHD mortality rate. Unfortunately, the average decrement in serum cholesterol in this study was only 9 % while the mean serum cholesterol at entry was 247mg/100ml. What would the result have been with an entry mean cholesterol of 300, a 20 or 30 % serum cholesterol decrement and intervention for other risk factors? It is hoped that some of the answers will be forthcoming from the trials still in progress.

Should the practising physician use lipid-lowering drugs, in view of the preceding considerations from primary and secondary prevention trials? It needs to be stressed that management of an individual patient is far different from blind therapy in a trial. Under clinical care conditions, the patient is selected because of marked hyperlipidaemia, the treatment is individualised, the serum cholesterol response is assessed and the treatment modified if the results are inadequate.

Perhaps this amounts to a rationalisation and lipid-lowering drugs really offer no benefit for the patient! The authors consider that the positive results of intervention studies already available cannot be ignored, but they do stress the need for selective use of lipid-lowering drugs in patients most likely to benefit. It would seem that lipid-lowering drugs do reduce morbidity in patients with pre-existing CHD and that their use is indicated in such patients with hyperlipidaemia, *provided a substantial decrement in lipids is produced*. In regard to primary prevention, the use of lipid-lowering drugs seem justifiable on an empirical basis, provided again that a substantial decrement in lipids is produced. If serum lipids do not show substantial falls towards the desirable range, then the therapy should be discontinued.

Synopsis

The benefits of risk factor intervention will be greatest in subjects with multiple risk factors. The pathological evidence for significant regression of advanced atherosclerosis in man is meagre. Hence, intervention should be commenced as early as possible, aiming to achieve maximum modification but without causing harm.

Undisputed benefit has been demonstrated following intervention for cigarette smoking and high blood pressure, even in patients with pre-existing atherosclerosis. Cholesterol-lowering diets are associated with a lower CHD mortality rate and a trend towards lower total mortality. This benefit is not observed in the elderly (> 65 years) or in patients with previous myocardial infarction.

The use of lipid-lowering drugs in patients with pre-existing CHD is associated with lower non-fatal re-infarction rates, if a substantial fall in serum lipids occurs. No clear effect on mortality has emerged in this patient group. The long term benefits of lipid-lowering drugs in subjects with hyperlipidaemia, who are still free of CHD, remain uncertain although effects on CHD morbidity are beginning to emerge, without change in CHD mortality. Such treatment is at present justifiable on an empirical basis.

References

1. Armstrong, M.L.; Warner, E.D. and Connor, W.E.: Regression of coronary atheromatosis in rhesus monkeys. Circulation Research 27: 59-67 (1970).
2. Barndt, R.; Blankenhorn, D.H.; Crawford, D.W. and Brooks, S.H.: Regression and progression of early femoral atherosclerosis in treated hyperlipoproteinemic patients. Annals of Internal Medicine 86: 139-146 (1977).

3. Gordon, T.; Kannel, W.B.; McGee, D. and Dawber, T.R.: Death and coronary attacks in men after giving up cigarette smoking. A report from the Framingham Study. Lancet 2: 1345-1348 (1974).
4. Mulcahy, R.; Hickey, N.; Graham, I.M. and MacAirt, J.: Factors affecting the 5 year survival rate of men following acute coronary disease. American Heart Journal 93: 556-559 (1977).
5. Veterans Administration Co-operative Study Group on Antihypertensive Agents. Journal of the American Medical Association 213: 1143-1152 (1970).
6. Berglund, G.; Wilhelmsen, L.; Sannerstedt, R.; Hansson, L.; Andersson, O.; Sivertsson, R.; Wedel, H. and Wikstrand, J.: Coronary heart disease after treatment of hypertension. Lancet 1: 1-5 (1978).
7. Whyte, H.M.: Potential effect on coronary heart disease morbidity of lowering the blood cholesterol. Lancet 1: 906-910 (1975).
8. Committee of Principal Investigators: A co-operative trial in the primary prevention of ischaemic heart disease using clofibrate. British Heart Journal 40: 1069-1118 (1978).
9. National Heart Foundation of Australia Committee on Diet and Heart Disease: Dietary fat and coronary heart disease: A review. I. Diet in the prevention of coronary heart disease and some pathogenetic aspects. Medical Journal of Australia 1: 575-579 (1974).
10. Report of a Working Group on: Diet and coronary heart disease. Australian Acadamy of Science Report Number 18 (1975).
11. Miettinen, M.; Turpeinen, O.; Karvonen, M.J.; Elosuo, R. and Erkki, P.: Effects of cholesterol-lowering diet on mortality from coronary heart disease and other causes. A 12 year clinical trial in men and women. Lancet 2: 835-838 (1972).
12. Dayton, S.; Pearce, M.L.; Hashimoto, S. and Dixon, W.J.: A controlled clinical trial of a diet high in unsaturated fats in preventing complications of atherosclerosis. Circulation 40 (Suppl. II): 1-63 (1969).
13. Joossens, J.V.; Vuylsteek, K.; Brems-Heyns, E.; Carlier, J.; Claes, J.; De Backer, G.; Graffar, M.; Kesteloot, H.; Kornitzer, M.; Lequime, J.; Pannier, R.; Raes, A.; Van Houte, O.; Vastesaeger, M. and Verdonk, G.: The pattern of food and mortality in Belgium. Lancet 1: 1069-1072 (1977).
14. Palmer, J.; Woodhill, J.; Leelarthaepin, B.; McGilchrist, C. and Blacket, R.: The Sydney Diet Heart Study: final result. Australian and New Zealand Journal of Medicine 7: 549 (1977).
15. Report of a Research Committee to the Medical Research Council: Controlled trial of soya bean oil in myocardial infarction. Lancet 2: 693-699 (1968).
16. National Heart Foundation of Australia: Dietary fat and coronary heart disease: A review. III. A community programme. Medical Journal of Australia 1: 663-668 (1974).
17. Coronary Heart Disease. A progress report, 1976. National Heart Foundation of New Zealand (1976).
18. Select Committee on Nutrition and Human Needs, United States Senate: Dietary goals for the United States. (U.S. Government Printing Office, Washington 1977).
19. Study Group of Physicians, Newcastle-upon-Tyne: Trial of clofibrate in treatment of ischaemic heart disease. British Medical Journal 4: 767-775 (1971).
20. Scottish Society of Physicians: Ischaemic heart disease: A secondary prevention trial using clofibrate. British Medical Journal 4: 775-784 (1971).
21. Krasno, L.R. and Kidera, G.J.: Clofibrate in coronary heart disease. Effect on morbidity and mortality. Journal of the American Medical Association 219: 845-851 (1972).
22. Coronary Drug Project Research Group: Clofibrate and niacin in coronary heart disease. Journal of the American Medical Association 231: 360-381 (1975).
23. Carlson, L.A.; Danielson, M.; Ekberg, I.; Klintemar, B. and Rosenhamer, G.: Reduction of myocardial re-infarction by the combined treatment with clofibrate and nicotinic acid. Atherosclerosis 28: 81-86 (1977).
24. Dorr, A.E.; Gundersen, K.; Schneider, J.C.; Spencer, T.W. and Martin, W.B.: Colestipol hydrochloride in hypercholesterolemic patients — effect on serum cholesterol and mortality. Journal of Chronic Diseases 31: 5-14 (1978).

25. The Multiple Risk Factor Intervention Trial: A national study of primary prevention of coronary heart disease. Journal of American Medical Association 135: 825-827 (1976).
26. WHO European Collaborative Group: An international controlled trial in the multifactorial prevention of coronary heart disease. International Journal of Epidemiology 3: 219-224 (1974).
27. Wilhelmsen, L.; Tibblin, G. and Werko, L.: A primary prevention study in Gothenburg, Sweden. Preventive Medicine 1: 1-2 (1972).
28. Sturdevant, R.A.L.; Pearce, M.L. and Dayton, S.: Increased prevalence of cholelithiasis in men ingesting a serum cholesterol lowering diet. New England Journal of Medicine 288: 24-27 (1973).

Chapter IV

Diagnosis of Hyperlipidaemia

1. Who to Measure

There are 5 main groups of individuals who deserve consideration for lipid testing:
1) Those with symptomatic vascular disease
2) Those with upper abdominal pain and/or pancreatitis
3) Those with metabolic conditions associated with secondary hyperlipidaemia
4) Those with other cardiovascular risk factors
5) Asymptomatic individuals.

1.1 Symptomatic Vascular Disease

Hyperlipidaemia was present in 31 % of myocardial infarct survivors in one study, while this prevalence rose to 60 % in males under 40 years and females under 50 years of age [1]. While the merits of intervention in these patients may be debatable, there is a strong case for precise aetiological diagnosis. Moreover, the diagnosis of significant hyperlipidaemia may lead to diagnosis of affected relatives still free of vascular disease.

1.2 Acute Abdominal Pain

Acute upper abdominal pain, with or without pancreatitis, is an important indication for the assessment of plasma lipids. Whole blood examined 5 to 10 minutes after sampling will have a characteristic 'cream of tomato soup' appearance if marked

Table I. Metabolic conditions with secondary hyperlipidaemia

Condition	Class of hyperlipidaemia[1]	Reversible with specific treatment of condition
Obesity	Hypertriglyceridaemia	Yes
Diabetes	Hypertriglyceridaemia	Yes
Hypothyroidism	Combined hyperlipidaemia (occasionally type III)	Yes
Oestrogen therapy	Hypertriglyceridaemia	Yes
Alcoholism	Hypertriglyceridaemia	Yes
Nephrotic syndrome	Combined hyperlipidaemia	No
Chronic renal failure	Hypertriglyceridaemia	No
Renal transplantation	Combined hyperlipidaemia (Occasionally hypercholesterolaemia)	No
Liver disease	Hypertriglyceridaemia	Yes
Dysglobulinaemia	Hypertriglyceridaemia	Yes

1   Only the most common association is represented.

hypertriglyceridaemia is present. The separated plasma will also be extremely turbid under these conditions.

1.3 Metabolic Conditions Associated with Secondary Hyperlipidaemia

A variety of metabolic diseases often have associated lipid abnormalities (table I). Several of these conditions are themselves linked with cardiovascular disease. The presence of these diseases should be excluded before initiating a lipid-lowering regimen.

Diabetes Mellitus

Individuals with diabetes have an increased prevalence of hypertriglyceridaemia. Recent studies have also documented low HDL levels in these patients which respond positively to appropriate therapy [2]. Lipid analyses may thus provide one index of diabetic control.

Renal Diseases

The nephrotic syndrome and chronic renal failure are frequently accompanied by hyperlipidaemia, combined hyperlipidaemia in the former instance and usually hypertriglyceridaemia in the latter [3]. In view of the concurrent presence of other risk factors such as hypertension and cigarette smoking, hyperlipidaemia should be diagnosed as part of total disease management. After renal transplantation, hypertriglyceridaemia is frequently normalised although hypercholesterolaemia may be a persisting problem.

Hypothyroidism

Hypothyroidism is often characterised by combined hyperlipidaemia [4]. Treatment with thyroxine should reverse this lipid abnormality.

Oestrogens and Oral Contraceptive Use

Oestrogens and oral contraceptives may in certain situations induce hypertriglyceridaemia [5]. The pathological significance of this is uncertain at present since in some individuals oestrogen may actually increase HDL levels [6]. These changes are reversible over a period of months and it may be necessary to suspend these agents in instances of certain complications, such as abdominal pain.

Alcohol

In susceptible individuals alcohol ingestion may induce hypertriglyceridaemia of moderate to severe degree. This is completely reversible by cessation of alcohol intake.

Other Disorders

A miscellaneous group of disorders may lead to abnormalities in lipid metabolism. These disorders include liver diseases, dysglobulinaemias and certain autoimmune conditions.

1.4 Individuals with Other Cardiovascular Risk Factors

Data presented in earlier chapters have stressed the interaction of the various risk factors. Patients who suffer from hypertension or obesity, or those smoking cigarettes, merit a measurement of serum lipids. This would apply particularly to subjects with a family history of hypercholesterolaemia.

1.5 Asymptomatic Individuals

The results of lipid-lowering therapy previously discussed suggested that primary prevention of atherosclerosis offered the only real hope of reducing cardiovascular mortality. Measurement of lipids in asymptomatic individuals provides such an opportunity for primary prevention. If a community-wide measurement of lipids is to be undertaken, either in screening clinics or by individual practitioners, this needs to be part of a total risk factor profile analysis. In this way subjects at greatest risk can be identified and intervention suggested.

2. Diagnosis and Classification of Hyperlipidaemia

The diagnosis of hyperlipidaemia should comprise an initial measurement of serum lipids, followed by a secondary analysis in those subjects with borderline or elevated values. One reason for this secondary lipid analysis is that cholesterol and triglyceride assays are technically difficult and sometimes even the best laboratories may have measuring errors of 5 to 10%. The follow-up examination in selected cases might also include an evaluation of the lipoprotein phenotype.

Blood samples should be analysed initially for both cholesterol and triglyceride concentrations. Irrespective of whether triglycerides are a primary or secondary risk factor, knowledge of the levels of both lipids provides a rational basis for management. An assessment of the need for treatment then usually can be made on the basis of cholesterol and triglyceride levels alone. Routine measurement of phospholipids and free fatty acids will add little further information in the diagnosis of hyperlipidaemia.

Approximately 45 to 65mg/100ml (1.17-1.70mmol/litre) of total serum cholesterol is transported in the HDL fraction. This contribution is probably only of diagnostic importance when total serum cholesterol *is less than 300mg/100ml*. In this circumstance a separate quantitation of HDL cholesterol might provide a better assessment of risk.

Occasionally, the translation of the serum lipid profile into a hyperlipoproteinaemic type can provide a more precise evaluation of the lipid transport defect involved. Hyperlipoproteinaemias represent abnormal accumulations of different lipoproteins. This may be due either to overproduction, defective removal or a combination of these problems. The aetiologies of these disorders may be specific genetic defects, underlying metabolic disorders, or environmental factors. Despite such heterogeneous aetiologies, lipid transport disorders may be expressed as one of only a few morphological or phenotypic expressions. Classification of the hyperlipidaemias in terms of the particular lipoprotein classes affected provides the basis of the popular lipoprotein phenotyping system of Fredrickson and Lees [7].

This phenotyping system, while usefully identifying lipoprotein transport disorders, eventually leads to the assumption that each phenotype represents a single disease in terms of its pathophysiology, whereas this is clearly not the case. For this reason there is now a trend away from lipoprotein phenotyping and this is reflected in the subsequent discussion. Here, hyperlipidaemia will be classified as hypertriglyceridaemia, hypercholesterolaemia and combined hyperlipidaemia, though related for ease of reference to the Fredrickson or WHO classification (table II). The hyperlipidaemias are also discussed in terms of their pathophysiology, a classification suggested by Brunzell et al. [8].

Table II. Classification of hyperlipidaemia

Class	Approximate lipid levels (mg/100ml)	Stored serum	Lipo-protein abnor-mality	Fred-rickson type	Pathophysiology
Hypertrigly-ceridaemia (normal cholesterol)	160-1000	Uniformly turbid	↑VLDL	IV	VLDL overproduction, removal defect
Massive hypertri-glyceridaemia (variable cholesterol)	> 1000	Creamy supernatant	Chylo-microns	I	LPL[1] deficiency
		Creamy supernatant, turbid intranatant	Chylo-microns + ↑VLDL	V	LPL functional defect, VLDL overproduction
Hyperchole-sterolaemia (normal triglyceride)	> 240	Clear	↑LDL	IIa	LDL removal defect, LDL and cholesterol over-production
Combined hyper-lipidaemia	Chol. > 240 Trig. > 160	Clear to turbid	↑LDL + ↑VLDL	IIb	VLDL and LDL overproduction and removal defects
			Beta-VLDL	III	Defect in VLDL catabolism to remnants

LPL = Lipoprotein lipase.

2.1 Hypertriglyceridaemia

Type I hyperlipoproteinaemia is characterised by the presence of massive chylomicron triglyceride in the fasting state. It is the creamy layer over a clear infra-natant plasma after 4°C storage which distinguishes this hyperlipidaemia from type V. The pathophysiological basis of the disorder is an inherited deficiency of lipo-protein lipase, the enzyme controlling lipoprotein triglyceride clearance. It is an extremely rare disorder presenting in childhood with eruptive xanthomata and acute abdominal pain.

A second genetic disorder characterised by massive hypertriglyceridaemia has only recently been identified [9]. This is due to a functional rather than an absolute lipoprotein lipase deficiency. The heritable defect has been identified as a deficiency of apo C-II, the endogenous apoprotein activator of lipoprotein lipase.

Type IV hyperlipoproteinaemia is due to elevated VLDL, where total triglyceride levels would range between 2 and 10mmol/litre approximately. Stored plasma is uniformly turbid without a chylomicron layer. Type IV hyperlipidaemia is the most common form of hypertriglyceridaemia. It may be familial but more commonly arises as a secondary hyperlipidaemia (table I). The pathophysiological basis for this disorder appears to be a heterogeneous picture, due either to overproduction of VLDL, as in carbohydrate induced hypertriglyceridaemia, alcoholism [10], or oestrogen therapy [11], or due to impaired function of the lipoprotein lipase-mediated removal system, as in chronic renal failure [12] and diabetes mellitus [13].

Another form of massive hypertriglyceridaemia is type V hyperlipoproteinaemia, characterised by the presence of chylomicrons and excess VLDL in fasting serum, by triglyceride values usually in excess of 10mmol/litre and by cholesterol values which may be normal or elevated. This syndrome represents a diverse metabolic picture, often secondary to obesity, diabetes or alcoholism, occasionally induced by oestrogens and rarely familial [14]. Overproduction of VLDL and saturation of removal mechanisms have been documented.

2.2 Hypercholesterolaemia

Type IIa hyperlipoproteinaemia is due to an elevation of cholesterol-rich LDL or beta lipoprotein. It may usually be identified without electrophoresis by the presence of elevated cholesterol levels, since most of the plasma cholesterol is transported as LDL cholesterol. This hypercholesterolaemia may be genetic in origin, secondary to disorders such as hypothyroidism or the nephrotic syndrome, or may be of uncertain aetiology, probably reflecting an interaction between dietary and undefined polygenic factors. The pathophysiological basis appears to be a combination of excessive production and defective catabolism of cholesterol [15]. In familial hypercholesterolaemia, the cellular defect has been identified as a deficiency in LDL surface receptors, which results in an inability to degrade LDL cholesterol and to suppress cholesterol synthesis [16]. Other disorders manifesting as type IIa hyperlipidaemia are more heterogeneous in their pathophysiology.

2.3 Combined Hyperlipidaemia

Combined hyperlipidaemia usually implies increased LDL and VLDL, that is type IIb hyperlipoproteinaemia. In practical terms its presence is suggested by an elevation in cholesterol and triglyceride values. These criteria alone do not distinguish type IIb from type III hyperlipoproteinaemia. However, type III is an extremely uncommon disorder and for practical diagnostic purposes it can be ignored in this context, unless palmar or tuberous xanthomata are present (*vide infra*). Type IIb hyperlipoproteinaemia is the phenotypic manifestation of a variety of defects which may include VLDL and LDL overproduction, with or without VLDL and LDL removal defects.

Type III hyperlipoproteinaemia is a rare form of combined hyperlipidaemia, strongly associated with premature coronary heart disease and with peripheral vascular disease. For these reasons intervention is particularly indicated in this condition. One is alerted to the possible existence of type III hyperlipoproteinaemia through the presence of palmar xanthomata or tuberous deposits over elbows and knees, particularly if these had 'melted away' with therapy in the past. The definitive diagnosis requires preparative ultracentrifugal analysis, followed by the demonstration of beta migrating VLDL and a ratio of VLDL cholesterol to plasma triglyceride greater than 0.3 [17]. The pathophysiological basis for this disease is an abnormal accumulation of intermediates in VLDL catabolism, often called intermediate density lipoprotein or IDL [18]. This disorder may be genetic but is occasionally seen in association with hypothyroidism or obesity.

Type V hyperlipidaemia may also be characterised by elevated levels of both cholesterol and triglycerides and could be considered a variety of combined hyperlipidaemia. However, this problem is predominantly one of chylomicron and VLDL metabolism with marked hypertriglyceridaemia. For this reason, it is considered in the hypertriglyceridaemia group.

2.4 Prevalence of Hyperlipidaemia

Relatively few truly representative cross-sectional assessments of the prevalence of hyperlipidaemia have been performed around the world. However a reasonable approximation of the community prevalence of these conditions may be obtained from data generated by risk factor screening programmes [19]. Examples of such data are presented for the Sydney Coronary Heart Disease Prevention Programme in table III, based on 13804 subjects, under 60 years of age, tested over 2 years. The definition of hyperlipidaemia used in this table is not a statistical one, but is based on purely arbitrary cut-off values. It is noted that the prevalence of hyperlipidaemia increases with age and triglyceride problems are much less common in women.

It is difficult to draw precise comparisons between these findings and those in other communities because of important differences in sampling, methodology and cut-off values. A number of studies in Australia [20, 21], Europe [22, 23] and the USA [24, 25] have produced broadly similar results to those in table III.

3. Sampling Considerations

Although cholesterol levels are not significantly altered by the ingestion of fat, triglyceride levels fluctuate widely. For this reason it is recommended that serum

Table III. Prevalence of hyperlipidaemia in subjects attending the Sydney Coronary Heart Disease Prevention Programme

Diagnosis	Males (%)		Females (%)	
	21-39 years (no = 2326)	40-59 years (no = 3868)	21-39 years (no = 1885)	40-59 years (5725)
Hypercholesterolaemia[1]	8.7	15.8	9.3	29.5
Hypertriglyceridaemia[2]	15.1	21.2	2.4	4.4
Combined hyperlipidaemia[3]	5.5	11.7	0.8	6.2
Totals	*29.3*	*48.7*	*12.5*	*40.1*

1   Cholesterol > 240mg/100ml, triglycerides < 160mg/100ml.
2   Triglycerides > 160mg/100ml, cholesterol < 240mg/100ml.
3   Cholesterol > 240mg/100ml, triglycerides > 240mg/100ml.

lipids be measured after a 12 to 14 hour overnight fast, a procedure which allows accurate assessment of a single blood sample. Subjects are allowed to take water during this fast. If a cholesterol reading alone is required, then fasting is not necessary.

Certain circumstances may lead to artifactual variation in apparent lipid values. Care must be taken to avoid venous stasis through prolonged tourniquet application. This may lead to a 5% elevation in plasma lipid levels. Ideally, sampling should be performed in the same position, either sitting or recumbent, since a reduction in lipid levels can be induced by the expansion of plasma volume with assumption of the reclining position.

Attention should be given to the presence of intercurrent illness and/or concurrent medication when interpreting serum lipids. In particular, myocardial infarction is known to be followed by an acute fall in cholesterol levels which may not return to normal for several months [26]. Surgery, major trauma, respiratory infections and gastrointestinal upsets can also result in reduction in lipid levels. Serum lipid levels normally rise during the second and third trimesters of pregnancy [27] and this should be considered in interpreting lipid values. Many drugs may also increase serum lipids as well as alter lipoprotein concentrations. These include diuretics [28], β-blockers [29], oestrogens and oral contraceptives [5], as well as corticosteroids [30]. It is of interest in terms of cardiovascular risk that β-blockers lower HDL levels [29] while oestrogens may induce a rise [6].

Blood samples should be immediately chilled to 4°C if lipoprotein fractionation or other sophisticated tests are contemplated. Routine cholesterol and triglyceride assays, however, are not adversely affected by exposure of blood samples to room temperature for several hours. For practical purposes, the concentration of cholesterol and triglycerides in serum or plasma is identical. The decision whether to use serum or anti-coagulated plasma for analysis is usually an arbitrary one, but consideration should be given to the assays to be undertaken and to the anticipated storage of samples. If it is intended to freeze samples, then the use of serum is preferred to avoid the formation of clots. Lipoprotein analysis and other more complex measurements require the presence of an anti-oxidant such as EDTA.

4. Analytical Considerations

4.1 Cholesterol Estimation Methodologies

One aim of lipid analysis for screening purposes is a rapid diagnosis without loss of accuracy or precision. Any reader who is interested in choosing between cholesterol measuring procedures should consult a recent review of this subject by Zak [31]. There are two principal categories of cholesterol measuring methods in use by analytical laboratories. The first involves organic extraction of serum, hydrolysis of cholesterol esters to free cholesterol and colourimetric determination of free cholesterol by chemical reactions of the Liebermann-Burchard or ferric chloride variety. The second principal category comprises methods using enzymatic procedures to isolate free cholesterol and to convert it to detectable endproducts.

The Liebermann-Burchard and ferric chloride reactions are traditional cholesterol measuring methods which have been automated to provide low material cost as well as speed and accuracy. The Liebermann-Burchard reaction measures free cholesterol after reaction with a sulphuric acid/acetic acid/acetic anhydride mixture, while the ferric chloride method differs in that it uses a sulphuric acid/acetic acid/ferric chloride endpoint. The latter method has the advantage of increased sensitivity and stability of colour development relative to the Liebermann Burchard reaction. The Liebermann-Burchard reaction is also particularly susceptible to interference from bilirubin in jaundiced serum. The ferric chloride reaction on the other hand suffers interference from the presence of bromide, which is used to increase serum density during ultracentrifugation. This ion is readily removed with an ion exchange resin. All non-enzymatic methods are nonspecific and may measure other sterols but in human serum these do not usually make a significant contribution.

Enzymatic cholesterol determination is theoretically simpler and more specific than either of the chemical assays. The most serious limitation of the enzymatic method is the large number of potential inhibitors present in normal and pathological serum [31]. Furthermore, non-human reference sera may upset a quality control programme with this method.

4.2 Triglyceride Estimation Methodology

A recent international study comparing serum triglyceride methodology in 10 laboratories using 25 different methods emphasised the potential variability in triglyceride determination [32]. All current reliable methods depend upon hydrolysis of triglycerides and subsequent analysis of free glycerol. As with cholesterol, the procedures fall into two categories, chemical or enzymatic.

Chemical methods utilise a nonspecific alkaline hydrolysis and as a result must have a means of removing phospholipids, a potential source of glycerol, as well as glucose. This readily achieved with zeolite or alumina. Endpoint determination is fluorometric, requiring scrupulous attention to glassware, tubing and reagents to avoid interference.

Enzymatic triglyceride analysis is relatively specific but is subject to some limitations. This method will include measurement of the level of free glycerol in serum, as well as of triglyceride glycerol. This is not usually an appreciable error. Again there may be potential enzyme inhibitors in serum.

Selection of a laboratory for lipid analysis should include consideration of internal and external standardisation and appropriate attention to quality control assessment. A good laboratory should be able to achieve inter-assay co-efficients of variation of less than 10%.

4.3 HDL Cholesterol Determination

The recommended methods for HDL cholesterol determination involve either ultracentrifugal isolation of HDL or precipitation of all non-HDL cholesterol, prior to cholesterol analysis. Quantitation of HDL cholesterol through direct lipoprotein electrophoresis is not yet widely accepted. For routine laboratories, the only practical method is precipitation. There are three methods for selective precipitation of LDL and VLDL. They use heparin/manganese chloride, phosphotungstic acid/magnesium chloride or dextran sulphate/magnesium chloride [33]. The methods are similar in principle but only the latter method has been used successfully with enzymatic cholesterol methods [34].

Heparin/manganese precipitation is the most widely used procedure at present, but suffers from the potential for incomplete precipitation of LDL and VLDL. A modification has been introduced recently by the Lipid Research Clinic programme which has reduced this tendency, but care should be taken to avoid this source of error [35]. Phosphotungstic acid/magnesium precipitation appears to be more reliable and has been found to agree extremely well with the heparin/manganese procedure.

The physiological range of HDL cholesterol is 45 to 65mg/100ml (1.17-1.70mmol/litre) approximately. In addition, extremely small departures from the norm, changes as small as 3 to 4mg/100ml (0.08-0.18mmol/litre), may signify an important change in CHD risk. The accuracy and precision required to measure reliably such small differences in this low range is probably not yet available in every routine laboratory. For this reason, and because of the difficulty in interpretation of HDL levels, the authors do not recommend an assessment of HDL cholesterol for routine diagnostic purposes.

4.4 Lipoprotein Analysis

Lipoprotein electrophoresis using paper, cellulose acetate or agarose provided the basis for the WHO lipoprotein phenotyping system. The technique is a useful diagnostic tool for type III hyperlipoproteinaemia, but it is a qualitative procedure and only semi-quantitative at best. It is not necessary to perform routine lipoprotein electrophoresis in all patients to reach a final diagnosis.

Ultracentrifugal isolation is the only widely practised method of isolation of plasma lipoproteins. Readers seeking further practical details on preparative ultracentrifugation are referred to standard texts on the subject [36]. Analytical ultracentrifugation is a powerful tool for detecting and quantitating subtle changes in lipoprotein density and composition.

5. The Interpretation of Lipid Results

Hyperlipidaemia is associated with cardiovascular risk in a continuous relationship (chapter II, 1.1). There appears to be no clear threshold lipid value, below which protection is assured. The question as to what constitutes significant hyperlipidaemia is therefore a difficult one. The purely statistical approach labels those with lipid levels above the 95th percentile for age and sex as being hyperlipidaemic. These individuals are certainly those most likely to develop atherosclerosis. After consideration of the high average lipid levels in the whole population, relative to those in cultures with a much lower prevalence of heart disease, the appropriate lipid threshold should perhaps be much lower than the statistically determined norm.

It is recommended that adults under 55 years of age with cholesterol levels greater than 6.5mmol/litre (250mg/100ml) and/or fasting triglyceride levels greater than 2.0mmol/litre (180mg/100ml) should be *considered* for treatment. Lower limits are indicated in children, although there is no uniform agreement on what they should be. Lipid levels in the aged should be viewed extremely conservatively.

Synopsis

Measurement of serum lipids is indicated in patients with symptomatic vascular disease, in patients with abdominal pain and/or pancreatitis, in patients with other cardiovascular risk factors and in patients with metabolic diseases known to influence lipid metabolism. Asymptomatic individuals may also benefit from lipid testing if this is coupled with total risk factor assessment, accompanied by appropriate follow-up measures.

Hyperlipidaemia is usefully classified on the basis of its dominant lipid problem, either as hypercholesterolaemia, hypertriglyceridaemia or combined hyperlipidaemia. These disorders may be due to specific genetic defects, or to underlying metabolic problems such as obesity, diabetes or alcoholism, or they may be of uncertain aetiology.

Estimation of total plasma cholesterol and triglycerides alone is frequently suffi-cient to allow appropriate therapeutic measures to be undertaken. The qualitative technique of lipoprotein electrophoresis occasionally provides further useful informa-tion for the clinician. Quantitation of HDL cholesterol may in certain circumstances provide an additional and more precise assessment of cardiovascular risk. The in-terpretation of serum lipids must take into account age and sex, and the presence of other risk factors, intercurrent illness and concurrent medication.

References

1. Goldstein, J.L.; Hazzard, W.R.; Schrott, H.G.; Biermann, E.L. and Motulsky, A.G.: Hy-perlipidemia in coronary heart disease. I. Lipid levels in 500 survivors of myocardial infarction. Journal of Clinical Investigation 52: 1533-1543 (1973).
2. Calvert, G.D.; Graham, J.J.; Mannik, T.; Wise, P.H. and Yeates, R.A.: Effects of therapy on plasma-high-density-lipoprotein cholesterol concentration in diabetes mellitus. The Lancet 2: 66-68 (1968).
3. Ibels, L.S.; Simons, L.A.; King, J.O.; Williams, P.F.; Neale, F.C. and Stewart, J.H.: Studies in the nature and causes of hyperlipidaemia in uraemia, maintenance dialysis and renal transplantation. Quarterly Journal of Medicine 44: 601-614 (1975).
4. Lasser, U.L.; Burns, B. and Solar, S.: Type III hyperlipoproteinemia secondary to hypothyroidism; in Schettler and Weizel (Eds) Atherosclerosis III, p.621-625 (Springer-Verlag, Berlin 1974).
5. Wallace, R.B.; Hoover, J.; Sandler, D.; Rifkind, B.M. and Tyroler, H.A.: Altered plasma lipids associated with oral contraceptive or oestrogen consumption. The Lancet 2: 11-14 (1977).
6. Bradley, D.D.; Wingerd, J.; Petitti, D.B.; Krauss, R.M. and Ramcharan, S.: Serum high-density-lipoprotein cholesterol in women using oral contraceptives, estrogens, and progestins. The New England Journal of Medicine 299: 17-20 (1978).
7. Fredrickson, D.S. and Lees, R.S.: A system for phenotyping hyperlipoproteinemia. Circulation 31: 321-327 (1975).
8. Brunzell, J.D.; Chait, A. and Bierman, E.L.: Pathophysiology of lipoprotein transport. Metabolism 27: 1109-1127 (1978).
9. Breckenridge, W.C.; Little, J.A.; Steiner, G.; Chow, A. and Poapst, M.: Hypertriglyceridemia associated with deficiency of apolipoprotein C-II. The New England Journal of Medicine 298: 1266-1273 (1978).
10. Lieber, C.S.: Effects of ethanol upon lipid metabolism. Lipids 9: 103-116 (1974).
11. Glueck, C.J.; Fallat, R.W. and Scheel, D.: Effects of estrogenic compounds on triglyceride kinetics. Metabolism 24: 537-545 (1975).

12. Ibels, L.S.; Reardon, M.F. and Nestel, P.J.: Plasma postheparin lipolytic activity and triglyceride clearance in uremic and hemodialysis patients and renal allograft recipients. Journal of Laboratory and Clinical Investigation 87: 648-658 (1976).

13. Pykalistu, O.J.; Smith, P.H. and Brunzell, J.D.: Determinants of human adipose tissue lipoprotein lipase. Effect of diabetes and obesity on basal and diet-induced activities. Journal of Clinical Investigation 56: 1108-1117 (1975).

14. Simons, L.A.; Williams, P.F. and Turtle, J.R.: Type V hyperlipoproteinaemia revisited: Findings in a Sydney population. The Australian and New Zealand Journal of Medicine 5: 210-219 (1975).

15. Simons, L.A.; Reichl, D.; Myant, N.B. and Mancini, M.: The metabolism of the apoprotein of plasma low density lipoprotein in familial hyperbetalipoproteinemia in the homozygous form. Atherosclerosis 21: 283-298 (1975).

16. Goldstein, J.L. and Brown, M.S.: The low-density lipoprotein pathway and its relation to atherosclerosis. Annual Review of Biochemistry 46: 897-930 (1977).

17. Albers, J.J.; Warnick, G.R. and Hazzard, W.R.: Type III hyperlipoproteinemia: A comparative study of current diagnostic techniques. Clinica Chimica Acta 75: 193-203 (1977).

18. Chait, A.; Hazzard, W.R.; Albers, J.J.; Kushwaha, R.P. and Brunzell, J.D.: Impaired very low density lipoprotein and triglyceride removal in broad beta disease: Comparison with endogenous hypertriglyceridemia. Metabolism 27: 1055-1066 (1978).

19. Simons, L.A. and Jones, A.S.: Coronary risk factor screening and long term follow-up. Year 1 of the Sydney Coronary Heart Disease Prevention Programme. Medical Journal of Australia 2: 455-458 (1978).

20. Welborn, T.A.; Murphy, B.P.; Stewart, A.J.; Fullerton, R. and Finch, P.S.: Prevalence of cardiovascular risk factors including fasting serum triglyceride levels in the Cunderdin Health Survey of 1971. Medical Journal of Australia 2: 199-204 (1976).

21. Nestel, P.J.; Quinlivan, N. and Roxburgh, H.: Possible usefulness of screening for hyperlipidaemia. Medical Journal of Australia 2: 203-205 (1977).

22. Lewis, B.; Chait, A.; Wootton, I.D.P.; Oakley, C.M.; Krikler, D.M.; Sigurdsson, G.; February, A.; Maurer, B. and Birkhead, J.: Frequency of risk factors for ischaemic heart disease in a healthy British population with particular reference to serum lipoprotein levels. Lancet 1: 141-146 (1974).

23. Leren, P. and Haabrekke, O.: Blood lipids in normals. Acta Medica Scandinavica 189: 501-504 (1971).

24. Wood, P.D.S.; Stern, M.P.; Silvers, A.; Reaven, G. and von der Groeben, J.: Prevalence of plasma lipoprotein abnormalities in free-living population of the Central Valley, California. Circulation 45: 114-126 (1972).

25. Luepker, R.V.; Kent Smith, L.; Gillis, A.; Kochman, L.; Warbasse, R. and Sherwin, R.: Serum lipid levels in a clerical workforce. Journal of Chronic Diseases 30: 547-555 (1977).

26. Tibblin, G. and Kramer, K.: Serum lipids during the course of an acute myocardial infarction and one year afterwards. Acta Medica Scandinavica 174: 451-455 (1963).

27. Williams, P.F.; Simons, L.A. and Turtle, J.R.: Plasma lipoproteins in pregnancy. Hormone Research 7: 83-90 (1976).

28. Ames, R. and Hill, P.: Elevation of serum lipid levels during diuretic therapy of hypertension. American Journal of Medicine 61: 748-757 (1976).

29. Tanaka, N.; Sakaguchi, S.; Oshige, K.; Niimura, T. and Kanehisa, T.: Effect of chronic administration of Propranolol on lipoprotein composition. Metabolism 25: 1071-1075 (1976).

30. El-Shaboury, A.H. and Hayes, T.M.: Hyperlipidemia in asthmatic patients receiving long term steroid therapy. British Medical Journal 2: 85-86 (1973).

31. Zak, B.: Cholesterol methodologies: A review. Clinical Chemistry 23: 1201-1214 (1977).

32. Carter, T. and Wilding, P.: Factors involved in the determination of triglycerides in serum: an international study. Clinica Chimica Acta 70: 433-447 (1976).

33. Burstein, M.; Scholnick, H.R. and Morfin, R.: Rapid method for the isolation of lipoproteins from

human serum by precipitation with polyanions. Journal of Lipid Research 11: 583-595 (1970).

34. Finley, P.R.; Schifman, R.B.; Williams, J. and Lichti, D.A.: Cholesterol in high density lipoprotein: use of Mg^{+2}/dextran sulfate in its enzymic measurement. Clinical Chemistry 24: 931-933 (1978).

35. Albers, J.J.; Warnick, G.R.; Wiebe, D.; King, P.; Steiner, P.; Smith, L.; Breckenridge, C.; Chow, A.; Kuba, K.; Weidman, S.; Arnett, H.; Wood, P. and Schlagenhaft, A.: Multi-laboratory comparison of three heparin-Mn^{2+} precipitation procedures for estimating cholesterol in high density lipoprotein. Clinical Chemistry 24: 853-856 (1978).

36. Lindgren, F.T.; Jensen, L.C. and Hatch, F.T.: The isolation and quantitative analysis of serum lipoproteins; in Nelson (Ed) Blood Lipids and Lipoproteins: Quantitation, Composition and Metabolism, p.181-274 (Wiley Interscience, New York 1972).

Chapter V

The Management of Hyperlipidaemia

1. General Perspectives

Proper management of hyperlipidaemia entails lowering of elevated serum lipids by substantial amounts, preferably into the 'desirable' range if that can be achieved without causing untoward effects. If one begins with an extreme degree of hyperlipidaemia, then a compromise result might have to be accepted.

In adult subjects, it is suggested that a plasma cholesterol in excess of 6.5mmol/litre (250mg/100ml) or a triglyceride value in excess of 2.0mmol/litre (180mg/100ml) requires consideration for treatment. Plasma cholesterol concentration in teenagers probably should not exceed 5mmol/litre (195mg/100ml) but this is less certain. If any of these situations is accompanied by other major risk factors, then the case of intervention is further strengthened.

In the presence of advanced or disseminated atherosclerotic disease, or in subjects more than 60 years of age, it may not be advisable to begin intervention, although the patient himself may already have begun this with dietary modification. Patients with hyperlipidaemia and other risk factors who have submitted to reconstructive vascular surgery constitute a special group. Although no data are available about the benefits of lipid-lowering therapy in these patients, there is a strong empirical case for intervention.

2. Lipoprotein Changes with Therapy

The classical objective with lipid-lowering therapy is attainment of normal lipid levels. Such an approach takes no account of shifts in individual lipoprotein classes. Traditional lipid-lowering diets or drugs usually reduce the level of LDL. In treat-

Table I. Effects[1] of individual lipid-lowering therapies on lipids and lipoproteins

Treatment	Cholesterol	Triglycerides	VLDL	LDL	HDL
Usual cholesterol lowering diet	↓	0, ↓	0	↓	↓
Vegetarian diet	↓	0	0	↓	↓
Low calorie, reducing diet	↓	↓	↓	0, ↓	0, ↑
Clofibrate	↓, 0	↓	↓	↓(↑)	0, ↑
Cholestyramine	↓	0(↑)	0(↑)	↓	0
Nicotinic acid	↓	↓	↓	↓	↑
Probucol	↓	0	0	↓	↓
Sitosterol	↓	0	0	↓	↓

1 ↑ = increase, ↓ = decrease, 0 = no change.

ment terms, should one be at all concerned with changes induced in HDL? No firm answer to this question is available yet.

From a theoretical standpoint, one might become concerned if the effect of lipid-lowering therapy was to increase the ratio of LDL to HDL. In other words, an absolute fall in HDL cholesterol level by itself caused by treatment may not be all important, nor might an apparent increase in HDL be as beneficial as it would seem. The dominant effects of therapy on lipoprotein levels are summarised in table I. The present state of the art does not require a frequent estimation of lipoprotein levels during treatment; total lipids will usually suffice.

3. The Seven Point Guide to Management

1) Decide what you will accept as desirable lipid values and which patients will require treatment.

2) Exclude clinically and/or biochemically any underlying metabolic factors, such as obesity, diabetes, alcoholism, hypothyroidism, chronic renal failure, nephrotic syndrome, oral contraceptive medication, and liver disease. These will require specific therapy.

3) All overweight subjects should attempt reduction to ideal body weight, irrespective of the type of lipid abnormality.

4) At ideal or stable weight, hypercholesterolaemic patients should be switched to a cholesterol-lowering diet, low in cholesterol and saturated fats and enriched with polyunsaturates. A similar diet would be prudent in hypertriglyceridaemic subjects but is less essential.

5) Many patients will have satisfactory plasma lipids within 6 weeks with the dietary therapy described above. In more resistant cases therapy should be supplemented with clofibrate 1g twice daily. This will have a modest effect in hypercholesterolaemia and will be more effective in hypertriglyceridaemia. (The new drug probucol may eventually find application at this point in the treatment plan, in a dose of 500mg twice daily).

6) Persistent cases of hypercholesterolaemia usually yield to treatment with cholestyramine 16 to 24g/day (2-3 sachets twice daily before meals). Patients unable to tolerate cholestyramine may be able to take an alternative resin colestipol, in an equivalent sachet dosage.

7) Very resistant cases of hypercholesterolaemia and/or hypertriglyceridaemia usually respond to nicotinic acid in a dose of 3 to 6g/day after meals. Combination drug therapy is sometimes indicated in these patients.

It should be noted that this approach to treatment does not require lipid typing but does require the reader to diagnose whether the picture is a dominant cholesterol or triglyceride problem, or perhaps a mixed hyperlipidaemia. Points 2 to 7 will now be discussed at length, and some illustrative case histories given.

3.1 Secondary Hyperlipidaemia

The prescription of diet or lipid-lowering drugs is likely to be an unsuccessful and certainly illogical way of treating hyperlipidaemia when this is secondary to underlying metabolic problems such as those listed under point 2 above. To test for any of these conditions is simple and inexpensive. Occasionally primary hyperlipidaemia may co-exist with one of these situations and this will become apparent in due course.

3.2 Removal of Excess Weight Is Important

Many obese subjects have normal serum lipid levels. However, many subjects with hyperlipidaemia are overweight to some extent. Lipids should be re-measured at ideal or stable body weight following a period of successful weight reduction. At this time hypertriglyceridaemia will be significantly improved to the point of normal levels, or occasionally to the point of a residual but mild hypertriglyceridaemia. This may then suggest the need for subsequent drug therapy.

Until recently it was felt that hypercholesterolaemia responded less impressively to weight reduction. Recent work suggests that some hypercholesterolaemic patients will respond to weight reduction and this should not be overlooked [1]. In all cases of dietary therapy, the medical practitioner would be well served to seek the collaboration of a dietitian.

3.3 The Cholesterol-lowering Diet

In non-overweight patients, or in those who have completed a course of weight reduction, the standard cholesterol-lowering diet becomes the cornerstone of medical therapy. In practice, one should not simultaneously offer a formal low cholesterol and low calorie diet. This combined diet severely restricts the choice of foodstuff and results in poor compliance. The particular choice of diet is a matter of priority and this must be carefully explained to the patient.

The usual cholesterol-lowering diet is one with a low intake of cholesterol and saturated animal fats, together with some replacement by polyunsaturated fats. The cholesterol intake should be less than 300mg/day, the ratio of P:S (polyunsaturated to saturated fats) should be at least 1.0 and the fat calories in the diet should be about 30% of total, distributed equally between polyunsaturated, mono-unsaturated and saturated. This diet no longer includes an unlimited consumption of polyunsaturates. The layman has been persuaded that polyunsaturates are 'good for the heart' no matter what the circumstance. This is certainly not true in the presence of obesity. With a cholesterol-lowering diet it is essential that the patient avoids extremes of intake. Once again, a consultation with the dietitian would transmit these purely chemical recommendations into instructions that the patient can easily follow, while maintaining a completely balanced diet.

Proper adherence to this diet should produce a 10 to 20% reduction in serum cholesterol level within 2 to 6 weeks. It is unlikely that the response will alter very much after 6 weeks, unless there is a change in compliance. It needs to be stressed to the patient that this dietary therapy is lifelong. Repeat lipid measurement should be made approximately every 6 weeks until satisfactory results have been achieved, and thereafter perhaps yearly. Considering that most cholesterol problems in the community are of a mild degree, this approach will have 'controlled' the majority of patients.

Hypertriglyceridaemia may improve with a cholesterol-lowering diet to a limited extent. However, alternative dietary approaches such as weight reduction remain the mainstay of management. Isocaloric carbohydrate restriction was once highly recommended in the management of hypertriglyceridaemia, on the assumption that the problem was carbohydrate induced. This is probably true in a minority of cases

Table II. Drug therapy in hyperlipidaemia

Drug	Hypercholes-terolaemia	Hypertrigly-ceridaemia	Combined hyperlipidaemia
Clofibrate (1g twice daily)	Yes	Yes	Yes
Cholestyramine	Yes	No	Only in combination
Colestipol (2-3 sachets twice daily)	Yes	No	with another drug
Nicotinic acid (1-2g 3 times a day)	Yes	Yes	Yes
Probucol (500mg twice daily)	Yes	No	?

but universal application of this approach has proved disappointing in non-over-weight subjects. In cases of massive hypertriglyceridaemia, pancreatitis and/or abdominal pain which are not associated with obesity, diabetes or alcoholism, the use of an extremely low fat intake (10-15% of total calories) may prove very effective in eliminating chylomicronaemia and abdominal pain. This diet is assisted by the use of medium-chain triglyceride oil, which does not require the formation of chylomicrons during absorption.

In the absence of a weight problem or other causes underlying the hyper-triglyceridaemia, one has little option but to consider lipid-lowering drug therapy as an alternative to diet.

3.4 Drug Therapy

Inevitably a proportion of patients will not have responded satisfactorily to diet-ary measures. These patients become candidates for lipid-lowering drug therapy. This should not become a casual decision, but one taken after some reflection, after re-measurement and after discussion with the patient.

It is the habit of some doctors to prescribe lipid-lowering drugs at the time of initial diagnosis, as though this were a limited or temporary course of treatment. This practice is to be deprecated. The reader is reminded of the degree of uncertainty associated with the benefits of this therapy, of the need for lifelong treatment, of the potential for serious side effects and of the heavy financial burden on the community. Despite these largely negative considerations however, many patients will and should be commenced on this type of drug therapy.

Table II summarises the indications for each drug according to the dominant type of hyperlipidaemia.

Clofibrate

Since publication of the findings of the WHO European clofibrate trial, some doctors have been reluctant to use clofibrate because of potential toxicity and apparently insufficient heart disease prevention. The present authors have formed the view that a significant reduction in heart disease morbidity results with clofibrate therapy and that the risk of potentially lethal toxicity may be non-existent. Despite results to the contrary, it is possible that a reduction in the CHD mortality rate might occur with clofibrate therapy under appropriate circumstances. These considerations do suggest the need for a degree of conservatism, such as treating selected patients only, demanding a substantial serum lipid decrement and readiness to suspend therapy if this does not result.

60 to 70 % of clofibrate-treated patients will exhibit a significant fall in plasma cholesterol or triglycerides. Clofibrate predominantly reduces elevated VLDL and hence its main effect is on triglycerides. In adults, the usual dose is 1.5 to 2g/day and it is effective in a twice daily regimen. The daily dose of 2g should not be exceeded.

The mode of action of clofibrate is not clear. It is an absorbable drug known to produce many metabolic effects, including an increase in lipoprotein removal, reduction in cholesterol synthesis and an increase in the excretion of cholesterol via the biliary and faecal routes. This latter action probably accounts for its potential for gallstone formation, through the production of lithogenic bile. An excess incidence of gastrointestinal diseases including neoplasms has been described in one large trial with clofibrate, but not in other trials (chapter III, 6.1).

Nausea and fluid retention have been reported occasionally with clofibrate but this is usually a temporary effect. Clofibrate is bound to serum albumin and caution should accompany its use in hypo-albuminaemic states, e.g. nephrotic hyperlipidaemia. Renal failure is also a relative contraindication to its use. Both these clinical settings will predispose to the occurrence of a reversible myopathic syndrome, characterised by muscle pains, weakness and cramps with the use of clofibrate; this reaction also occurs in apparently healthy individuals, but it is excessively rare and no real cause for concern.

Clofibrate potentiates the action of warfarin and extreme care should be taken to monitor the prothrombin time. The dosage of warfarin necessary to produce a given depression of the prothrombin time may need to be halved.

Cholestyramine

Cholestyramine resin is an effective cholesterol-lowering agent in the dose range 16 to 24g of base per day (corresponding to 4-6 sachets per day). Therapy is initiated with 3 to 4 sachets per day and may be increased up to 6 sachets per day if the response is inadequate. There is little benefit to be gained from a higher dose. Like clofibrate, cholestyramine may be taken twice daily. Serum cholesterol may fall by 25 to 30 % with this treatment. Its main effect is to reduce serum cholesterol and LDL levels, and it has no capacity to reduce triglyceride levels. Occasionally cholestyramine will actually increase triglyceride levels while cholesterol levels are falling.

Cholestyramine is a non-absorbable anion-exchange resin and this explains its principal side effects, namely disturbance of gastrointestinal function. Some patients complain of nausea but more commonly of constipation or firm stools. A little advance warning and the use of a faecal softener is often sufficient in these cases.

Cholestyramine interrupts the enterohepatic circulation of bile salts in the body. To compensate for this the liver cells convert more cholesterol to bile salt, ultimately resulting in a fall in plasma cholesterol concentration. A compensatory but usually lesser increase in endogenous cholesterol synthesis also results. Entrapment of bile salts by cholestyramine is not complete and it is unusual to experience fat malabsorption with the recommended dosage (see chapter I, 4.3).

Colestipol

Colestipol resin is a relatively new anion-exchange resin which is similar in most practical respects to cholestyramine. There are individual patients who are unable to tolerate cholestyramine because of gastrointestinal side effects and they may be managed with colestipol. Colestipol is dispensed in 5g sachets and the recommended dose is also 4 to 6 sachets per day, taken twice daily.

Nicotinic acid (niacin)

Nicotinic acid is a useful reserve drug in the treatment of hypercholesterolaemia, hypertriglyceridaemia or mixed hyperlipidaemia. It is a potent suppressor of LDL and VLDL levels in most hyperlipidaemic states. The severity of side effects accompanying its rapid absorption restricts its wider use.

Nicotinic acid is a peripheral vasodilator and will produce marked skin flushing at the beginning of therapy. This can be minimised by using a small dose at first. One suggested regimen is:

0.25g 3 times daily for 3 days,
0.5g 3 times daily for 3 days,
0.75g 3 times daily for 3 days, and then
1g 3 times daily.

Some resistant patients will require larger doses — between 3 and 6g/day. Tolerance to the flushing reaction usually develops after a few days at constant dosage. However, it is essential that all patients be warned that some degree of flushing, erythema or pruritus will occur at the beginning of therapy.

With nicotinic acid treatment, gastric irritation is occasionally troublesome and the drug should be taken after meals. Hepato-toxicity has been described as a rare complication. Nicotinic acid reduces serum lipid levels, probably through multiple mechanisms, including reduction of lipid and lipoprotein synthesis in the liver, partly due to reduction in the flux of substrate free fatty acids through plasma from adipose tissue to the liver.

Probucol

Probucol is the newest lipid-lowering drug to come into routine use. It is poorly absorbed from the gut, becomes concentrated in various lipid-rich tissues and persists in the body for a very long period of time. At an oral dosage of 500mg twice daily, it will predictably lower serum cholesterol levels by approximately 15%, with negligible influence on triglyceride levels. Minor gastrointestinal upsets, notably diarrhoea, have been reported but these are not especially troublesome. Several years' further use will be required for this new drug to find its correct place in routine lipid-lowering therapy [2].

Combination Drug Therapy

Combination drug therapy is sometimes indicated in more resistant patients on the basis of two drugs having complementary and/or synergistic modes of action. As previously stated, cholestyramine therapy is associated with an increase in cholesterol synthesis, potentially limiting its usefulness. The addition of an agent such as clofibrate or nicotinic acid, which is capable of reducing cholesterol synthesis, may be advantageous in this situation [3].

Alternatively, combination therapy with nicotinic acid and clofibrate has proved beneficial [4]. This has enabled the use of a smaller than otherwise dose of nicotinic acid, e.g. 3g/day nicotinic acid plus 2g/day clofibrate.

Duration of Therapy

Approximately 6 weeks of therapy is necessary with any drug to assess its efficacy. It is unusual to observe the onset of a therapeutic effect after this period unless there has been a change in drug compliance. Patients should be reminded that therapy with lipid-lowering drugs is potentially lifelong, as these conditions are controlled but not cured.

4. Illustrative Case Histories

A series of illustrative case histories derived from the authors' Lipid Clinic are presented. Most of these situations could be met in general practice. In addition examples of several uncommon situations are included.

4.1 Weight Reduction

Case 1

This was a 32-year-old male presenting with moderate hypertriglyceridaemia (type IV hyperlipoproteinaemia) in association with heavy cigarette smoking (fig. 1).

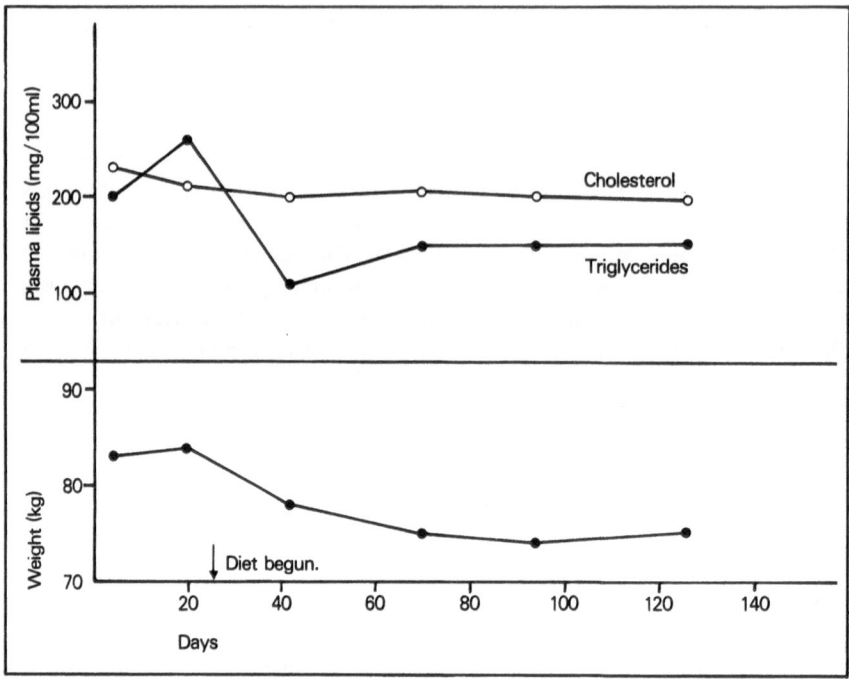

Fig. 1. The effects of weight reduction in a 32-year-old male patient with hyper-triglyceridaemia *(Case 1)*.

He was some 10kg in excess of his ideal body weight and, at routine family follow-up, was found to be hyperlipidaemic. He began following a 1,000 calorie reducing diet and had good weight loss. His triglyceride level averaged 230mg/100ml in the untreated state and fell rapidly to about 110mg/100ml when he entered the phase of negative caloric balance. As his weight began to stabilise his plasma triglyceride level began to rise slightly, but remained in the desired range. This is an example of normalisation of serum triglyceride through weight loss and weight maintenance.

Case 2

This patient was a 38-year-old female who presented with massive hyper-triglyceridaemia of the type V hyperlipoproteinaemia pattern (fig. 2). Her initial plasma triglyceride level exceeded 10,000mg/100ml. She had recently suffered from acute pancreatitis which had occasioned a laparotomy. She was about 20kg in excess of her ideal body weight at the time of presentation and was started on a 1,000 calorie reducing diet. She gradually reached ideal body weight over a period of 4 months. The plasma triglyceride level began to fall as soon as she had begun to lose weight. Although the weight loss continued for up to 4 months, the triglyceride level

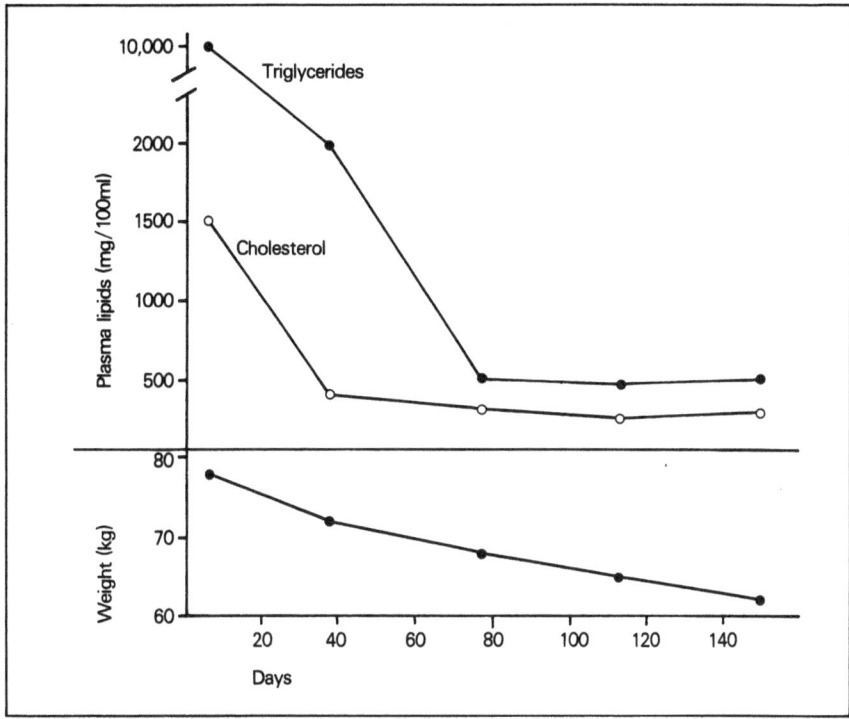

Fig. 2. The effects of weight reduction in a 38-year-old woman *(Case 2)*, with marked hypertriglyceridaemia (type V hyperlipoproteinaemia).

stabilised between 400 and 500mg/100ml. She maintained a similar weight over several more months while the triglycerides remained around 400mg/100ml. The plasma cholesterol level was 1,500mg/100ml at the beginning of treatment but this rapidly attained satisfactory levels. This patient clearly demonstrates a less severe, but persistent degree of hypertriglyceridaemia which was not corrected by the maintenance of ideal weight. She subsequently improved further with clofibrate therapy.

4.2 Diabetes and Alcohol

Case 3

A 54-year-old male presented because of marked hypertriglyceridaemia (type V hyperlipoproteinaemia) in association with coronary heart disease (fig. 3). There was a past history of congestive cardiac failure, diabetes mellitus and alcoholism. In hospital, he received various isocaloric diets and he maintained stable body weight. Withdrawal of alcohol led to improvement in plasma lipids but not in glucose

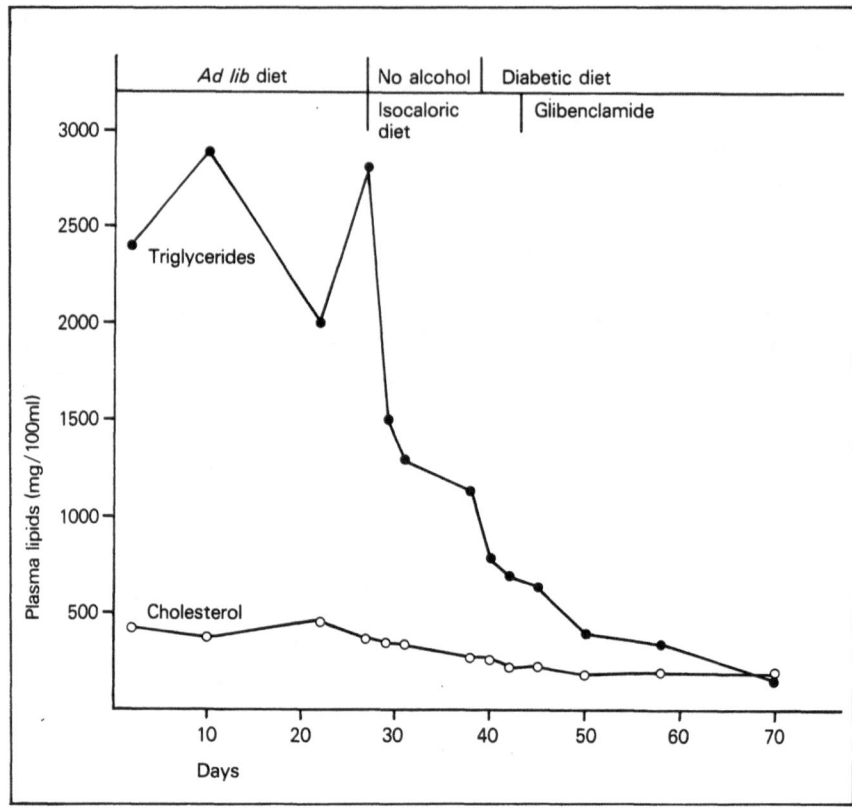

Fig. 3. The effects of diabetes management in a 54-year-old patient *(Case 3)* with marked hypertriglyceridaemia (type V hyperlipoproteinaemia).

tolerance. A diabetic diet plus an oral hypoglycaemic agent led to a rapid improvement in glucose tolerance and a gradual normalisation of plasma lipids over 4 weeks. This man is an example of mild diabetes not dependent on insulin, precipitating frank hyperlipidaemia.

Case 4

This patient was a 31-year-old man who presented with plasma triglycerides of 460mg/100ml (type IV hyperlipoproteinaemia) in association with a heavy alcohol intake (fig. 4). He was advised to totally abstain from alcohol which he successfully did. Within 3 days, his triglyceride levels had fallen to 145mg/100ml, remaining in the normal range over the next few months. Subsequently he returned to alcohol with a corresponding rise in triglyceride. This man demonstrates the important contribution of alcohol to some cases of hypertriglyceridaemia, the rapid nature of the response and the unfortunate liability to relapse. These patients in relapse often respond poorly to lipid-lowering drug therapy.

4.3 Marked Hypercholesterolaemia and Drug Therapy

Case 5

A 21-year-old male with hypercholesterolaemia (plasma cholesterol 8.3mmol/litre, triglycerides 1.5mmol/litre, type IIa hyperlipoproteinaemia) and smoking 25 cigarettes per day, was found during routine population testing (fig. 5). Clinical investigation, including measurements in close relatives, revealed no apparent cause for his hypercholesterolaemia. This was assumed to be primary in type and of uncertain cause. He was started on a cholesterol-lowering diet which lowered his cholesterol to 7.5mmol/litre. To obtain lower values clofibrate, 1g twice daily was introduced and follow-up cholesterol values from that time were less than 5.5mmol/litre. This case illustrates a straightforward response to diet and clofibrate.

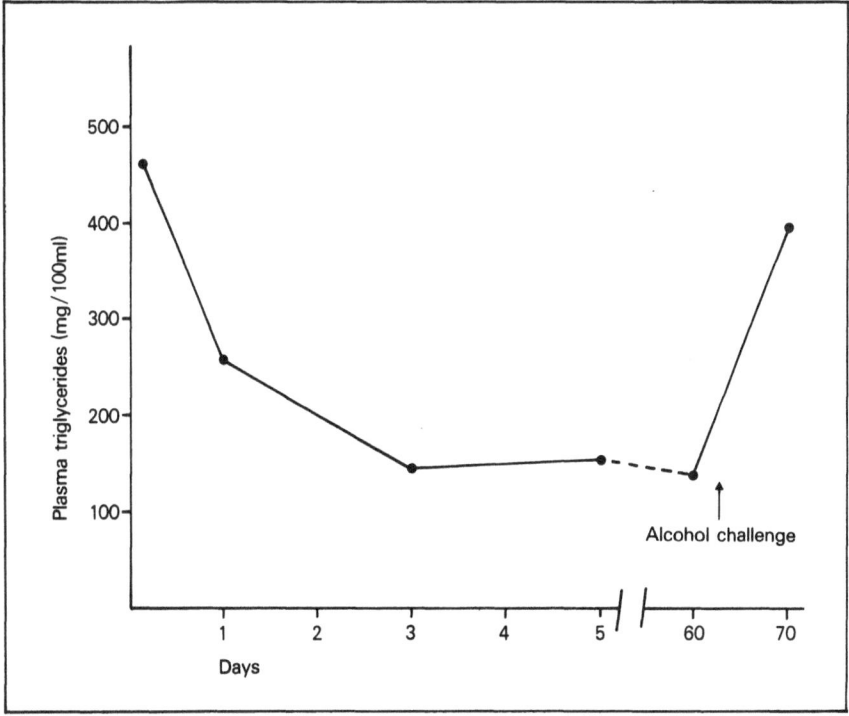

Fig. 4. The effects of alcohol withdrawal (zero time) and alcohol challenge in a 31-year-old male patient *(Case 4)* with hypertriglyceridaemia.

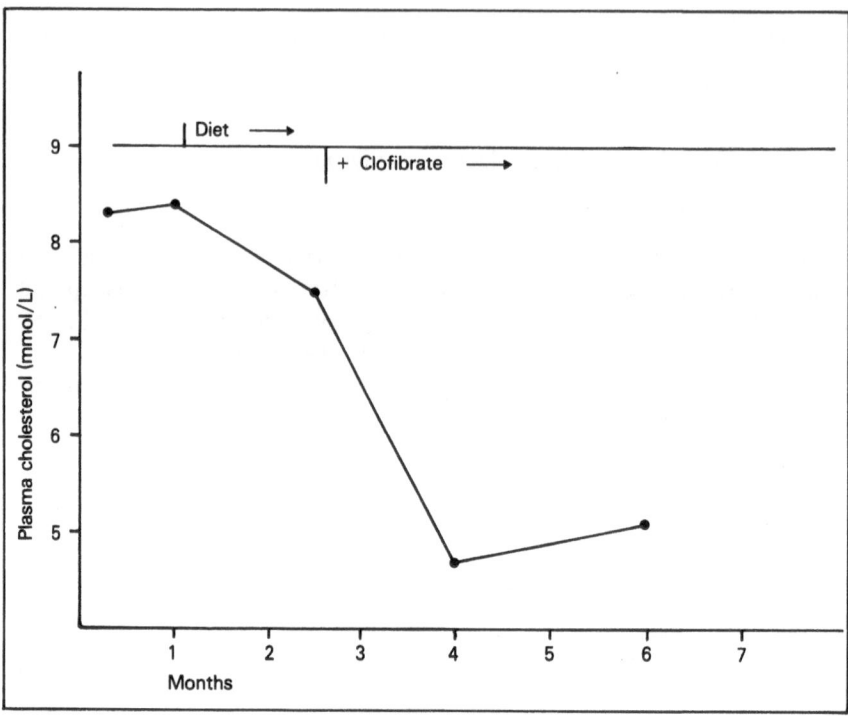

Fig. 5. The effects of diet and clofibrate in a patient with hypercholesterolaemia *(Case 5).*

An alternative and probably equally effective treatment might have been cholestyramine resin, 2 sachets twice daily.

Case 6

This patient was a 26-year-old female who presented with severe hypercholesterolaemia (cholesterol > 14mmol/litre, triglycerides 1.6mmol/litre, type IIa hyperlipoproteinaemia), diagnosed during lipid screening of the relatives of a man with familial hypercholesterolaemia and coronary heart disease (fig. 6). Clinical examination revealed the presence of a premature corneal arcus and xanthomata in the Achilles tendon bilaterally. A diagnosis of familial hypercholesterolaemia in the heterozygous form was made and the patient was offered a cholesterol-lowering diet for 1 month, pending the results of all her biochemical investigations.

A small drop in plasma cholesterol accompanied this diet to 13.0mmol/litre and she then started clofibrate at a dose of 1g twice a day. 4 weeks later her cholesterol was further improved at 10.1mmol/litre. Diet and clofibrate were supplemented with nicotinic acid 3g/day without further benefit (cholesterol 10.3mmol/litre). Nicotinic acid dosage was increased to 6g/day and over succeeding visits her plasma cholesterol stabilised below 7mmol/litre — a substantial fall in plasma cholesterol. This case demonstrates that patients may need extensive drug therapy, but that the principles of management remain unchanged even during combination drug therapy.

4.4 Type III Hyperlipoproteinaemia

Case 7

A 46-year-old male presented with combined hyperlipidaemia in association with severe peripheral vascular disease. One year previously he had undergone successful sapheno-femoral bypass grafting. He had xanthomata in the palmar skin creases, as well as over the elbows. His plasma cholesterol was 350mg/100ml and his triglycerides were 400mg/100ml. Lipoprotein electrophoresis and studies in the

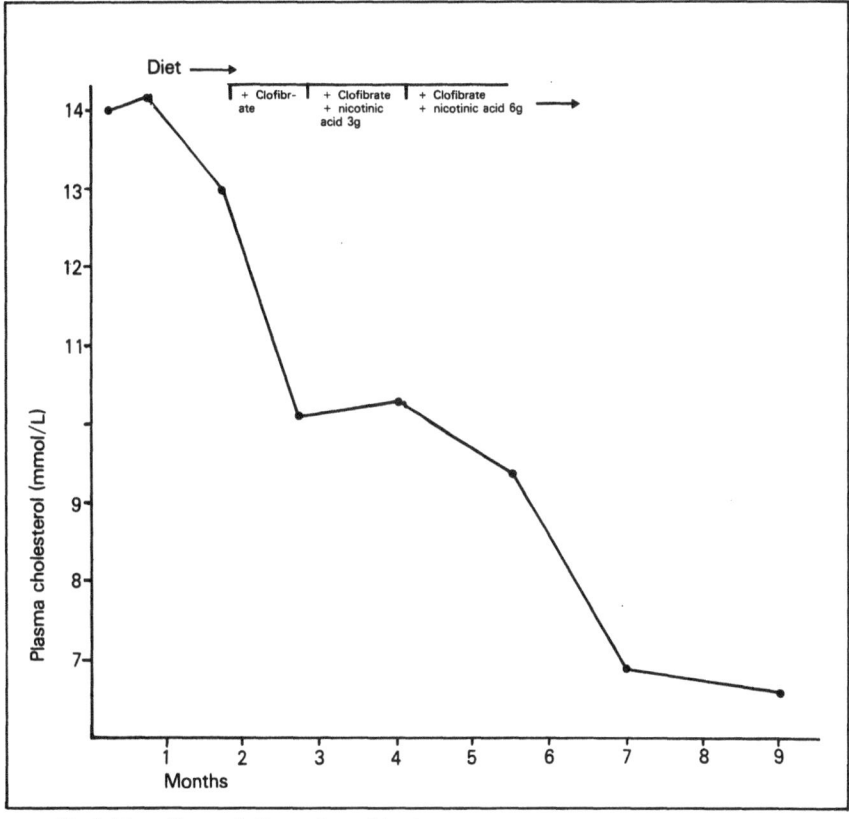

Fig. 6. The effects of diet and combination drug therapy in a patient with severe familial hypercholesterolaemia *(Case 6)*.

ultracentrifuge confirmed a diagnosis of the very rare type III hyperlipoproteinaemia (Broad Beta Disease). He was also 10kg over ideal weight.

Clofibrate, 1g twice daily, was started and this led to rapid resolution of his xanthomatous lesions. Unfortunately, a mild hyperlipidaemia persisted with a cholesterol value of 290 and triglycerides of 210mg/100ml. Subsequently he was able to lose his excess weight and normalise his lipids to a cholesterol value of 230 and triglycerides of 120mg/100ml. This case demonstrates the importance of weight control as well as the value of clofibrate in the rare type III abnormality. On lipid values alone, this patient might have been diagnosed as excess LDL plus VLDL, i.e. type IIb hyperlipoproteinaemia. However, the presence of palmar xanthomata is virtually pathognomonic of type III hyperlipoproteinaemia, although this may occur in primary biliary cirrhosis but with other characteristically diagnostic features.

4.5 Pancreatitis, Abdominal Pain and Hypertriglyceridaemia

Case 8

This patient, a female aged 26 years, presented with a 10-year history of recurrent upper abdominal pain associated with marked hypertriglyceridaemia (cholesterol 8mmol/litre, triglycerides 62mmol/litre, chylomicrons present in the fasting state, type V hyperlipoproteinaemia). Clinical examination revealed the presence of eruptive xanthomata over her elbows and buttocks. There were no underlying problems such as diabetes, obesity or alcoholism, and she was considered to be an example of primary hyperlipidaemia without familial involvement. She was started on a diet offering only 10% of the daily calories as fat. This diet was made more acceptable by supplementation with medium-chain triglyceride oil. Within a few days her daily attacks of abdominal pain had ceased and her xanthomata began to disappear. Over 4 weeks triglyceride levels fell to 10.6mmol/litre and eventually stabilised around 4mmol/litre. Plasma cholesterol stabilised in the range 4 to 5mmol/litre. From this point onwards, over a period of 2 years, she has been completely free of pain, except for occasional instances when she has chosen to eat a little more fat. This case illustrates the importance of strictly limiting the intake of total dietary fat in instances of abdominal pain and pancreatitis, where this is unaccompanied by other problems such as diabetes, alcoholism, or obesity.

5. Research Procedures; Unusual Therapies

Several unusual procedures have been investigated in the management of severely affected patients who may be resistant to conventional therapy. Repeated plasma exchange seems to be beneficial in the severely hypercholesterolaemic (but uncommon) homozygous patients with familial hypercholesterolaemia [5]. In the more numerous heterozygous subjects, the present authors have found the procedure no more effective than combination drug therapy, which is certainly more convenient [6].

Ileal by-pass surgery, whereby absorption of bile salts is prevented, has been used in a few centres [7]. Although this surgical procedure might avoid problems with compliance, cholestyramine therapy can be regarded as a pharmacological equivalent which is considerably easier and safer.

A number of older drugs have been used in the treatment of primary hyperlipidaemia but they should no longer be considered because of problems with toxicity, e.g. thyroxine, neomycin.

Synopsis

The management of hyperlipidaemia may be approached through the use of a seven point plan. Cases of secondary hyperlipidaemia should be diagnosed and treated appropriately. Dietary therapy is the cornerstone of medical treatment, a low calorie reducing diet for overweight patients and a cholesterol-lowering diet for hypercholesterolaemic patients who are not overweight. Many patients can be controlled by these measures alone but the therapy must be continued indefinitely.

A lesser number of patients will have persisting degrees of hyperlipidaemia which require drug therapy. Clofibrate is a useful drug for cholesterol or triglyceride problems, while the anion-exchange resins, cholestyramine and colestipol, are potent cholesterol-lowering drugs. The resins should not be used for essentially triglyceride problems. More resistant cases will respond to nicotinic acid therapy, while combination drug therapy is occasionally indicated. It should be stressed that lipid-lowering drug therapy must be continued indefinitely, provided a substantial serum lipid decrement has been achieved.

References

1.   Leelarthaepin, B.; Woodhill, J.M.; Palmer, A.J. and Blacket, R.B.: Obesity, diet and type II hyperlipidaemia. Lancet 2: 1217-1221 (1974).
2.   Heel, R.C.; Brogden, R.N.; Speight, T.M. and Avery, G.A.: Probucol: A review of its pharmacological properties and therapeutic use in patients with hypercholesterolaemia. Drugs 15: 409-428 (1978).
3.   Kane, J.P.; Tun, P.; Malloy, M.J. and Havel, R.J.: Heterozygous familial hypercholesterolemia: treatment with combined drug regimens. Clinical Research 26: 529A (1978).

4. Carlson, L.A.; Danielson, M.; Ekberg, I.; Klintemar, B. and Rosenhamer, G.: Reduction of myocar-
    dial re-infarction by the combined treatment with clofibrate and nicotinic acid. Atherosclerosis 28:
    81-86 (1977).
5. Thompson, G.R.; Lowenthal, R. and Myant, N.B.: Plasma exchange in the management of
    homozygous familial hypercholesterolaemia. Lancet 1: 1208-1211 (1975).
6. Simons, L.A.; Gibson, J.C.; Isbister, J.P. and Biggs, J.C.: The effects of plasma exchange on
    cholesterol metabolism. Atherosclerosis 31: 195-204 (1978).
7. Buchwald, H.; Moore, R.B.; Lee, G.B.; Frantz, I.D. and Varco, R.L.: Combined dietary, surgical
    and bile salt binding resin therapy in the treatment of hypercholesterolemia. Archives of Surgery 97:
    275-282 (1968).

Subject Index